JELLY DONUT DAYS
Fighting Breast Cancer, One Day at a Time

for Bridget & Family,
May your
jelly donut days
be few...
♡ MicHele

Michele Truran Brymesser

JELLY DONUT DAYS

Fighting Breast Cancer, One Day at a Time

Michele Truran Brymesser

Cover Photo by: Madelyne C. Brymesser

Bras, Boobs, and Biopsies

If this is too much information, read no further. The moment I found out that my mammogram didn't look good, I began writing. A friend told me that writing might help me cope. I'm trying to maintain my sense of humor. I hope my stories make you laugh on occasion. I choose happy. Prayers always appreciated. Let your faith be bigger than your fear. Warmly, Michele

Acknowledgements

With every attempt to write my acknowledgements, I found myself crying. So, I'll keep it simple. It is with my deepest, heartfelt appreciation, that I thank each and every one of you who have read my stories, laughed with me, cried with me, and reminded me that someday I would have my happy ending. May God richly bless all of your days, and may your faith always be bigger than your fear. May your lives be filled with the laughter of children, the warmth of family love, the fond memories of the past, and the hope of the future.

The Wisdom in this Book
Three jelly donuts in one day is *never* a good idea.

I dedicate this book to my
husband Mike and our children
Cody, Morgan, and Jordan

Without you, there would not be a happy ending.

In loving memory of my mom,
who always knew I would
someday write a book.

Yvonne Eileen Truran
February 22, 1935-August 5, 2001

When a Stranger Offers Comfort

Thursday, September 24

In the waiting room I sit in the tent-like gown, waiting for my mammogram result. I've done this seven times, and it never seems to get easier. While I can accept that my body type is obese, it seems that one could fit three of me in this oversize gown. I wrap it tightly around me because I can't even begin to figure out how it ties. Another lady walks in, same size as me *(I love how the gown color is what indicates size, as in — oh, she's a burgundy)*. Although she is smaller than me, she has managed to make the huge gown look somewhat like a wrap dress, and has it neatly tied in a bow. *I feel like the unmade bed.* We joke about the outdated magazines and try to find words to fill the awkward silence. And then…the tech comes to the door and calls my name. She calls me into the hallway, and I can't recall ever having been called out of the waiting room before. But yet, I think I've always been the only one in the waiting room. What follows is a bit of a blur — 2 cm. mass — need an ultrasound — please wait. When I walked back into the waiting room, I felt a little weak in the knees. Was it the lack of a healthy breakfast or just the overall dislike of being there? I can only remember telling the stranger my result and telling her repeatedly that I was so glad she was there, that had I been alone, I would have fallen into a puddle of tears. I remember telling her I was scared. I remember her offering words of comfort, yet I have no idea what she actually said to me.

The wisdom in this story: Angels usually tie their gowns neatly.

1

When it is Difficult to Talk

Friday, October 2

After what can only be described as a whirlwind week, many of my friends knew that I was scheduled for a biopsy. Everyone was praying, and wanted me to keep them updated. I think I knew that day that it was going to be cancer. The doctor said that *"based on the scans"* it didn't look good and that we would schedule an MRI *"just in case"* it was a cancer diagnosis. Cancer or not, the lump would need to be removed. An order for blood work was given and as I sat in the waiting room I felt numb. Beside me was my husband, my best friend…years of married togetherness. I wanted to reach out to him, but for what I think was the first time ever, I saw fear in his eyes. I picked up my cell phone. When I turned it on, the dinging of texts seemed unending. There were so many checking in, sending prayers, asking how things were going for me. I replied—to everyone. *I texted, and texted, and texted.* Out of the far corner of my eye, I could see my soul mate, someone I had loved since I was 18. He didn't seem to know what to say, and I didn't either. The silence was uncomfortable. For the first time ever, I didn't feel brave. In the arms of someone who knew me best, I should have been able to melt, but I didn't. In a world where we criticize teenagers for overuse of technology and social media, I was finding that I, too, could text words that I was unable to speak. In time, I will find a way to talk to my husband—just not yet. I think we both need to find our words.

The wisdom in this story: Put away the cell phone and hold the hand of someone near.

Victoria's Secret

Friday, October 2

My daughters LOVE Victoria's Secret. I remember when I bought my oldest daughter her first bra at that store, I made two comments:

#1. Don't tell your dad how much this bra cost.
#2. Don't ever let your dad put this bra in the dryer.

Me, well...um...I don't splurge in that department. Something functional. White, maybe nude. Occasionally black. Cheap brand. From the supercenter. Yep. So during the biopsy---the nurses asked me if I had a *"supportive"* bra. Sure. "Of course," I answered. Yes, my bra *(that my husband often mistakenly puts in the dryer),* is just fine. Then came the time for dressing my wound, with instructions to place an ice pack in the bra, and to wear the supportive bra for at least three days. At that moment, my slingshot looking brassiere from the supercenter didn't quite look *"supportive."*

The wisdom in this story: Always, always, shop at Victoria's Secret---and, buy PINK.

When Your Fingers are Numb

Friday, October 2

I'm a mom. I'm here at the football game in the pouring rain watching my girls cheer. Other moms are home in their fuzzy pajamas. But I am here, post biopsy — ice pack and all, never wanting to miss a thing my kids do.

The wisdom in this story: When your fingers are numb, your boob doesn't hurt.

I'm So Sorry You Have Cancer

Tuesday, October 6

As the doctor described, I received the news in a phone call from the nurse. I was specifically told in advance that I would be unable to ask questions. The nurse would basically say "yes, you have cancer" or "no, you don't." The details would come in the appointment to follow with the doctor. I wanted this call early, to find out before sitting face to face with the doctor. I was prepared for the news. I was okay with a yes or no. The details could wait. The words from the nurse were, *"there are some cancer cells."* Okay. There are some cancer cells. The doctor will tell me how to get rid of them. That's it. Get back to my classroom. Move on. I'm ready. After sharing the news with others, I got a text from a friend. It said, "Oh, sweet Michele...I am so sorry you have cancer. I give you my love and prayers and pray God's steady presence and peace upon you." While all of this should have brought me comfort, it was the first I had actually heard the words *"you have cancer."* That made it real.

The wisdom in this story: It's all in what you call it. I'm calling it "some cancer cells."

"How are you doing, Mom?"

Tuesday, October 6

My son. Mama's boy. He is 19. I can proudly say that this young man has never raised his voice to me, never slammed a door, and never shown an ounce of disrespect. To be honest, I sometimes wonder how I got so lucky. He, along with his 17-year-old sister and dad were all at the dentist when I received my news. They found out together. The littlest one would find out in her own time. Now back to this sweet young man, who still texts me his whereabouts regularly because he knows I worry. From the dentist office, he texts me this:

"How are you doing mom?"

Truthfully, I was crying—having a pity party in my classroom while my students were at their special classes. But I answered,

"Better than you, you're at the dentist."

He answered,

"Better be fine, because someone has to babysit my kids someday."

The wisdom in this story: Sometimes, things really are worse than going to the dentist.

"Do the kids know?"

Tuesday, October 6

Everyone asks if my kids *"know."* Of course they know. It's not a secret. We are a family. I will need their love and support and we will face this together. Someone asked if they're okay. I answered, "as expected." How is a kid supposed to act when they hear the news that mom has cancer? I don't know — but here's what I do know:

Age 19: I think he thinks I'm dying.

Age 17: She has the deepest look of concern on her face. She wants to talk, but seems scared.

Age 14: Sort of gets it. She is in her own happy bubble.

The wisdom in this story: I love happy bubbles.

They're Making Me Crazy

Wednesday, October 7

I am strong. I will beat this. It won't be fun. It will be difficult. But it will be okay. There are two people in my life who have cried more about this than I have. I understand that it is an emotional subject, but I'm feeling wrapped in prayer and able to say "it is what it is" and I'm ready to move forward. These people in my life — they mean well — but you can hear it in their voices. They tell me how awful this news is and how they just don't know what to say. They cry as they speak. *To be honest, it's a little hard not to laugh.* Through thick and thin, these are people I know I can always count on, people who will always be there for me. But they're making me crazy.

The wisdom in this story: I don't do drama.

Brave, Strong, Smart

Thursday, October 8

It is cancer. I am wrapped in prayer, loved by many. A Christopher Robin quote *(from our beloved Winnie the Pooh stories)* pretty much sums it up.

> *"You are braver than you believe,*
> *stronger than you seem,*
> *and smarter than you think."*
> *(AA Milne)*

Today was that kind of day. I needed to be brave *(although the doctor told me it was perfectly fine to cry)*; strong is what will help me get through the days ahead; and smart, well — some of the decision making today was in my hands. I pray I made a smart choice. So — here is where we are — and today is the day I launch an online journal page, something I hoped I'd never have to do. A Wide Excision (lumpectomy), Sentinel Lymph Node Biopsy, and possibly Axillary Dissection are scheduled for October 27. Radiation needed. Possible chemo. More details, stage, etc., will be available after my surgery. I have a post-op visit and radiation oncologist appointment on November 9. I meet with the medical oncologist on November 11. These big fancy medical words are for my doctor and nurse friends, and for those who have traveled this same journey themselves. For me, the big words are all a little overwhelming, and I promised myself to try not to search online. So, to keep things simple, it's all part of the big plan, the one I'm calling the BBP *(Brymesser Boob Project)*.

The wisdom in this story: If you don't laugh, you'll cry. And I KNOW the BBP made you laugh!

9

What Do I Need?

Thursday, October 8

You have all been so kind already. You have asked what I need: I don't need meals, my husband and kids cook. Housework, yep...they do that, too. Errands, my oldest daughter has a driver's license and my red card. I may need a red store chaperone...I don't think she realizes the direct correlation between my red card and my bank account. Well, maybe she does — but little sister certainly does not. So, what DO I need? I need you to continue to be yourselves around me. A smile is better than a question. I don't want this to be the big elephant in the room, but I don't really want to talk about it either. If you care to read and say a prayer, I would appreciate it. I need many partners in prayer.

The wisdom in this story: Live. Laugh. Love.

When You Get to Keep the Socks

Friday, October 9

My kids go to an indoor trampoline place. You jump a half
hour, sometimes an hour, and the best part of going is that
you get to keep *"the socks"* — neatly packaged, bright orange,
non-slip socks. I went for my MRI today. I wasn't the least bit
concerned about the procedure. I told my friend that I would
probably sleep. "You will NOT sleep," she said. She told me to
be prepared for lots of loud pounding noises. She forgot to tell
me to be prepared for an IV. She also forgot to tell me I would
be on my belly, not my back. When I entered the changing
room to yet another oversize gown *(I've proudly worn
burgundy, teal, now this one was a very faded floral)*, I smiled a
little to see a neatly packaged pair of light gray socks — like
trampoline socks. I changed quickly to be greeted by someone
that told me dye to the breast would go in through an IV in
my arm. *Hmm...this really isn't the quiet rest time I'd imagined.*
I'm terrible with an IV. No one can ever find a good vein. *(I
guess that doesn't look good for all that lies ahead).* So after they
found a reluctant spot in my hand for the IV, I plunked face
down on the table, ready to go. And then I heard them talking.
They didn't like the IV. There was no backflow of blood. *I
could never be a nurse.* They tried taping it, moving the tape,
wiggling it, and finally putting my hand on a pillow. "Let's
just try it," they said. *Oh, good heavens---try it?!? Try it means it
might not work, and does that mean that I would need to start all
over again?* I didn't ask. I did ask how long I would be "in
there" — she answered "about 15 minutes." She gave me
headphones and asked what music I liked, to which I replied
"anything but country." She gave me a little call bell to hold in
my hand. What followed seemed like an unending fifteen
minutes. I couldn't hear the music, and I really wanted to tell
her, *but I knew that wouldn't be an appropriate use of my call
button.* Yes, there was pounding — but then also the loudest,

most obnoxious beeping I've ever heard. It sounded a lot like our home security alarm, only magnified by ten, and right above my head. Then it was all over. They told me I did great. The IV did what it was supposed to do. I was dismissed to the changing room, my wrinkled clothing stuffed into the locker. There was a clothes hanger in there, but I doubt people really use them. I dropped out of the gown, and tore the socks off of my feet. I left them all behind and never looked back. From start to finish, I had been in this facility one hour. I had no desire to *"keep the socks."*

The wisdom in this story: The trampoline place has better socks.

Not Dying

Saturday, October 10

Someone thought I was dying because I have an online journal page. So in case you're wondering, I'm not even close to dying. This is just a small bump in my road. Online medical journal pages are for families who don't want to make dozens of emotional and time-consuming phone calls. It is a simple way of asking for prayers and keeping people informed. Online journal pages are for anyone, not just those with a terminal illness. After I shared my health concern with others, I was inundated with texts and social media messages. It was nearly impossible to remember with whom I communicated and those I neglected to remember to update. So I chose an online journal. So far, your comments make me smile. Keep commenting. *It's good for my ego.* I always wanted to be an author, and it seems my mother's wit and humor are sneaking into my words. Someone just told me I was *"laugh out loud funny."* That was perhaps the best therapy I needed. Love to all...and bless you for reading my stories.

The wisdom in this story: "I've still got a lot of fight left in me." (Rachel Platten)

When a Former Student Reaches Out

Saturday, October 10

Teachers never have favorites, yet there are always those who touch our hearts in a special way. I watched a sweet young six-year old girl grow through the grades, become my high school intern, and go off to college to pursue a degree in elementary education. She was an outstanding student and collegiate athlete, and earned a teaching position right out of college. She is a first-year teacher, and a blessing to all who are privileged to be in her class. To say I am proud is an understatement. She is just adorable...a blessing to me. She reached out to me with the most endearing, heartfelt text. Reading her words after diagnosis was one of the first times I cried.

"Hi! I just wanted to tell you that you were and always will be my favorite teacher, the one who changed my whole outlook on school and teaching. I can still imagine the wonderful things we did seventeen years ago like it was yesterday. You're one of the strongest women I know. Between teaching, being a mom, your hip, and just dealing with life, this little bump in life has nothing on you. I love you, my family loves you, and the world needs more people like you. I hope one day, I'll be a teacher just like you. I just wanted to send my love, magical healing powers, and for you to know you are never alone. Ever. I love you, Mrs. Brymesser." ~J

I replied.

M: I love you, J. May I share this on my online journal page?

J: Of course you can, I just subscribed to your page this morning. You're a fighter.

M: Yes! Feeling good. I love you.

14

J: I love you more.

The wisdom in this story: A teacher always loves her students. When that love is still reciprocated many years later it means the world.

When You Start the Day a Better Way

Sunday, October 11

Last Sunday, I was the first in my house to be awake. My husband and son went to work, my oldest daughter had homework to do before her job, and my youngest daughter *(like most teenagers)* was still in bed snuggled deeply under the covers. I planned to go to church solo, because I love the calming peace I feel in my life when I start my week with church. But, I came out to the kitchen, ate a jelly doughnut, and promptly crawled back in bed. Emotionally exhausted but not tired, what ensued was perhaps the biggest pity party I've ever had for myself. I did not emerge from the bedroom until noon, and was in a bit of a funk the rest of the day. This week was different. I went to church, my husband by my side, and spent the afternoon visiting with friends who are fighting their own battles. I took time to reflect on my doctor's words, to accept and feel satisfied with the plan that is before me. I sat outside for a bit and took a moment to appreciate the beautiful Fall foliage. God is good, all the time. All the time, God is good.

The wisdom in this story: While the occasional pity party is okay, it's best to avoid the jelly doughnut on Sunday mornings.

The Letter

Monday, October 12

After an emotionally exhausting long weekend, I will face my students tomorrow. I have guests coming—parent volunteers who play learning games and read stories to my class. I love having the parents visit, because I once so loved seeing my own young children in their elementary school environments. The parents and I exchange knowing glances and cute stories with one another, and I always try to find a brief moment to tell them how much I cherish their children. Tomorrow, I will be simply, Mrs. Brymesser—first grade teacher. Wednesday will be the same. However, Thursday will come, and my students will take a letter home to their parents. It will be neatly stapled to folders in an envelope marked confidential. My principal asked me to write a letter to parents explaining my impending absences. At first, I felt reluctant, but truly they deserve to know. So on Thursday, the parents will read the letter, and I will no longer simply be Mrs. Brymesser—first grade teacher. I will be Mrs. Brymesser—first grade teacher—the one with cancer. Now, before I have yet another pity party for myself, I need to tell you what my students currently believe. They think I have—allergies! You see, on the day after a particularly difficult doctor's appointment, I met with the children at circle time. As I occasionally suffer from seasonal allergies, I just happened to sneeze...three times. "Oh," I grumbled. "I still have allergies. These doctors need to help me get better." The class giggled. They love it when I'm dramatic and silly. A few days later, I told them I would be leaving at recess to go to yet another appointment. One sweet boy, small in stature, with the biggest brown eyes and dark curly hair came to my desk. "Good luck at the doctor," he said. Just as I smiled to myself about this young man being wise beyond his years, he said, "at least you didn't sneeze today."

Yes. It was a good day. I didn't sneeze. After Thursday, the parents and I will sadly exchange knowing glances of another kind. They will know my diagnosis, and reason for the absences that will follow. But in the world of six-year-olds, life is good — *especially if I don't sneeze.*

The wisdom in this story: There is always something good in each day.

So Hard to be Still

Friday, October 16

My youngest daughter is full of energy! She is the kid who doesn't pass through the kitchen, she cartwheels. She doesn't walk, she skips. She doesn't really ever sit still. *Ever.* Her body is in constant motion. Four and half weeks ago, *(coming down out of a 2-man cheerleading stunt)*, she sprained her ankle. Badly. The coach said she hardly cried. She came home on crutches, with the biggest ankle I've ever seen. Lots of swelling, lots of bruising---the x-ray somewhat inconclusive. The doctor said that her growth plates are closing, and sometimes a closing growth plate can resemble a fracture. Either way, treatment is the same....a boot. Some suggested an MRI. The doctor told us that all it would tell us was that she probably had several torn ligaments and some badly bruised bones. Yet still, the treatment would be the same…the boot. *Now you don't take a kid like Jordan and put her in a boot.* The recovery — the doctor told us that it would be "longer than it is short". It took awhile for me to comprehend that statement. He told me that some kids miss a whole season with an injury like hers. But he also told me that her return to cheerleading would be task-oriented rather than time-oriented. The more quickly she was able to return to each task *(walking, hopping, running, jumping, dancing, tumbling, and finally stunting)*, the more quickly she would be cleared to return to cheerleading. She wore the boot faithfully while at school, but went barefoot at home. Finally last week, a shoe would again fit. With only a brace, she began walking more comfortably, with only a slight limp. And then it was time to go shopping for the shoes...Homecoming shoes. It's doubtful that the athletic trainer or the doctor would approve the high heel sparkly shoes she chose, but you only have Freshman Homecoming once, and she was determined to make it work. She has walked around the kitchen in the sparkly heels for two days. Just last night, she put on her dancing-shoes and danced every dance number from last year's middle school musical. She had a feature leap in the actual musical. I had to gently remind her that a leap across the ceramic tile in her current condition probably wasn't a good idea. She persevered. She is almost *back*. She has been given permission to "walk the routine," and wants more than anything to have her spot on the mat back. It has been a journey for the little girl who doesn't sit still. She is a lot like me. I don't like to sit still. *Ever.* With the cancer journey ahead of me, I anticipate that the recovery will be "longer than it is short." I want to return to my routine daily tasks quickly. I pray that I have her determination, strength, and perseverance. I want to be *back.*

The wisdom in this story: Everyone needs a little bit of sparkle and some great dancing shoes.

One Size Never Fits All

Sunday, October 18

My oldest daughter is a Dairy Princess. Today, I had the privilege of accompanying three Dairy Princesses on their first State Royalty shopping trip! These delightful young ladies first met one another at a training seminar in July; they were crowned together at State Pageant in September; and now, they have a friendship fueled by their shared passion for the dairy industry and love of farm life. The girls, each unique in her own way, had a wonderful day together. Our favorite stop was a store that specializes in black and white clothing, *(of course the Holstein color theme always works with a princess sash!)* They wanted to coordinate outfits, without being too "matchy-matchy." The girls ranged in height from 5'2" to almost 5'10" *(yep, my kid was the shortest).* Their first choice of colors was black, gray, and maroon. One girl chose a fitted dress, another chose one more twirly, and yet the third enthusiastically stated, "I just love skirts." She paired her skirt with a dressy blouse and cardigan. Our program coordinator added her own flair with gorgeous maroon slacks paired with layered tops and a sparkly blazer. Individually, they looked terrific — but together, breathtaking. What a stunning, professional looking group of young women ready to educate our whole state about dairy! When it came time for shoes, one rocked the red pumps, another wobbled her way across the store, and the other openly stated that she preferred flats. As the mom, I was there to zip zippers, check sizes, find bargains, and tell them they looked great. Not once did I offer unsolicited advice. Not surprisingly, they all made equally appropriate choices for themselves. They knew their bodies and their comforts. They had learned to trust themselves, and when a fit felt right, they went with it. Which brings me to the next lesson in my cancer journey. Throughout the past several weeks, I've received more unsolicited advice than I care to remember. Yet there

21

have also been the people who are simply by my side to tell me I'm doing great. I've been faced with the decision to choose a lumpectomy with radiation and possible chemo, or choose a mastectomy. Choosing hasn't been easy. As with everything in life, there are pros and cons. I pray that I am making an appropriate choice for myself, and my doctor has guided me in stating that either choice is an equally curable method. I know my body and my comfort. I'm learning to trust myself and I'm going with it. The best thing friends can do for me now is show their continued support. A friend recently told me that I picked a *hell of a month* to be diagnosed. There is PINK everywhere. You can't escape it. While one girl likes skirts and the other prefers flats, I suppose it's okay to say that I've never really liked wearing pink. When I was a waitress at age sixteen, the uniforms were pink. The pink made my already very blue eyes look even more blue, and it seemed everyone noticed me. People were always complimentary in saying, "You have the most beautiful, big, blue eyes," but I was self-conscious and hated the attention the pink brought my way. Some people might think pink is a terrific color for me...but alone, it puts me out of my comfort zone. Yet, when so many pull together to wear pink, it is simply...breathtaking. It makes my big, blue eyes fill with tears.

The wisdom in this story: I'm gonna rock the PINK!

Sink or Swim

Monday, October 19

Today involved Pity Party #2, some not-so-good news, some GOOD news, some GREAT news, and another jelly doughnut.

Pity Party #2: I have decided that teaching is a *"sink or swim"* kind of profession. I've kept my head high above water for 26 years. I'm able to multitask, plan, and communicate effectively; I teach an incredibly challenging curriculum to six-year-olds; I'm able to make kids laugh; and most importantly, I believe that when most of them leave my classroom they love learning. They will become lifelong learners, and I pray that in some small way I've had a part in it. But lately I feel as if I've been sinking. It started before my diagnosis, *(so nope, we can't blame the cancer!)* Any current blog, newspaper article, or online post will tell you teachers all across the country are struggling. The cancer just makes the struggle even harder. I'm overwhelmed. Today after school, I was faced with more schoolwork than any newly diagnosed cancer patient should ever have to think about. So I did what most six-year-olds would do—I put my head down on my desk and I cried. I cried from four o'clock until almost five—when I realized that I had mail for the post office and some banking to do before closing time. I called my loving husband and cried some more. I finally out loud said what I've heard so many others say before. *"Cancer sucks,"* and my own, *"Sometimes school sucks, too."* Then, the day started to get better. My nurse *(so funny how I actually have my "own" nurse)*, called me.

The not-so-good news: My MRI revealed that the mass is larger than the 2cm expected. Under 2cm is easier to treat, over 2cm harder to treat. The doctor anticipated that it would measure below 2cm. It was larger, but only slightly. Not enough to change my course of treatment.

The GOOD news: My MRI revealed no other surprises...which I am assuming means no other visible cancers.

The GREAT news: My genetic test returned more quickly than usual. My BRCA1 and BRCA2 were both negative. Praise God.

And the jelly donut: My husband bought me a jelly donut. It seems as if jelly donuts and pity parties go together. My sister, who is also a teacher *(she's the best in the world)*, offered to write my lesson plans for me. I politely declined, but I was tempted.

The wisdom in this story: Sometimes school sucks. I need to buy my sister a jelly donut.

The Sunshine Lady

Thursday, October 22

When I was a small child, my mother was the neighborhood "Sunshine Lady." She was always sunshine to me, but the term Sunshine Lady meant she was a committee person in our very active neighborhood civic association. One of the responsibilities of the Sunshine Lady was to send cards, and I delighted in the beautiful assortment of greeting cards that mom stored in the antique secretary desk in our living room. Sometimes for fun, *(remember, I lived long before modern technology)*, I would spread all of the cards out across the floor and read them. I loved the embellished ones, the embossed ones, and the ones etched with what I truly believed was real silver. Some were funny *(probably adult humor far beyond my comprehension)* and some even in my young eyes looked serious and sad. One might think my love of cards at such a young age would make me a frequent visitor to the greeting card store. I love the greeting card store, but I seldom go there because to be honest, it's a bit of a daunting task. It's almost overwhelming—cards for every single occasion imaginable. I never have time to browse the way I like, so I avoid that store, instead grabbing a quick card here or there when I need one. Several years ago, I bought a whole box of sympathy cards. It seemed like everyone died that year. I used all the cards in a very short time period. I never bought another box of sympathy cards. So...while I'm fairly creative and thoughtful in gift giving, and love to recognize others, I'm terrible with cards. I simply don't buy them, or buy them and forget to send them. I have a sister-in-law and a cousin who never, ever neglect to send a card. One of my mom's dear friends always remembers my birthday and *always* gets the card to arrive in the mail on the exact day of my birthday. I often wonder how she does that each year. Since my diagnosis, my mailboxes at home and school have been overflowing. A sweet cousin who lost her own mom to breast cancer delivered a prayer shawl made by ladies at her church. Incredible friends just show up with meals, *(which my son seems to prefer to MY cooking).* The cards are coming, and coming, and coming. A letter from a friend I met in ninth grade reminded me of some of the wonderful times we have shared; another beautiful prayer shawl made by a retired teacher friend who now lives far away; a box full of everything pink and some much needed literature from a wonderful organization whose members are all breast cancer survivors); a beautiful card and pamper yourself items from our cheer boosters; and a box from a (cancer survivor) football mom with perhaps the most heartfelt letter I've ever read. Included with it were gifts from two of her friends who have been cancer patients. To say that I am appreciative is not enough. These people have reached deep within themselves and offered me HOPE. They have found ways big and small to brighten my days. They have warmed my heart. The days ahead are scary. Yes, I said it. I'm terrified. But I have faith in the wisdom of my doctor, and comfort in the arms of true friends. It's still just a little bump in the road. And when it's over, I'm going to the greeting card store.

The wisdom in this story: I have an incredible Sunshine Team.

Online Search

Thursday, October 22...again.

I promised myself I wouldn't online search. I searched.
Prayers for peace appreciated. My dear friend said it best —
Stay Properly Focused — SPF. It's all going to be okay.

The wisdom in this story: Don't search.

I don't know WHAT I am!

Saturday, October 24

Since diagnosis, I have a heightened sense of awareness of things around me. I notice everything. The skies seem prettier, the days seem longer, and things seem funnier. Somehow humor seems to be what is helping me stay strong. With this new sense of awareness, I can't help but notice the huge County Commissioner election signs that grace our roadways. I pay special attention to them, because both parties took quite an interest in my Dairy Princess daughter. One candidate invited her to a campaign fundraiser, and another candidate wanted to use her photo on their campaign literature. We politely declined both, because as Dairy Princess it is her role to represent only the farmers, and to be a friend and supporter of *all* people. So, as we drove home from the football game, our conversation turned to politics. My older daughter seemed to have a good grasp on which party was more conservative and which party was, as she called it, more free. I openly stated that I am a Republican. She sounded surprised that I would say so, and asked "isn't that supposed to be a *secret?*" I chuckled. Then I told her I've changed parties twice. I was once a teenage Republican *(because it was a cool group to join in school)*, switched to Democrat in college, and returned later in life to the Republican party. My husband shared his political affiliation, and moments later my youngest daughter *(four years younger than the voting age)* spoke out from the back seat..."I don't know WHAT I am!" I laughed out loud. Sometimes I don't know what I am either. As I face this cancer journey, people tell me I am a strong woman, yet sometimes I feel fragile. People tell me I am brave, yet often I feel terrified. Sometimes I can share my story easily, yet other times my eyes quickly fill with tears. This is all much, much harder than I'd ever imagined and it's only the beginning. It is certainly a journey of self-discovery. I've discovered that it's a good thing I'm a very busy person. I have a teaching job I love and adorable little ones who keep me busy — all day long. I have my own children who need me to be simply, Mom. I'm Mama B to some other pretty terrific teenagers who, without embarrassment, freely offer me hugs and knowing looks. It is in the quiet times that I fall apart. I feel a little helpless. My husband is there, trying to be brave, but I don't think he knows what he is either. So yes, last night was Pity Party #3. Today is a new day. I just sent the girls on a red card store run (*still no volunteers from y'all to be their credit-card chaperone*), and told them to get cash back for the donut shop. It seems it's another jelly doughnut kind of morning. But after noon today, my weekend schedule is packed. Everything will be okay. Really, it's okay to not know what I am — I'm a little mixed up bit of everything. To those who have already traveled this path — I know you understand.

The wisdom in this story: Life can never promise to always be happy.

Another Jelly Donut

Monday, October 26

What started as my first pity party and jelly donut story has turned into a joke among friends. My doctor performs surgery at two hospitals. The joke is that I selected the closer hospital because there is a donut shop next door. Truthfully, I selected the closer one *(even though all of my babies were born at the other one)* because it offered the first available surgery date. I feel like I'm in excellent hands there, and since it's outpatient, I won't be staying long and yes, I can still have my jelly donut. I had a fairly uncomfortable procedure today *(Sentinel Node Injection for you medical people out there)* and yes, we stopped for donuts on the way home. My donut was delicious and fresh, but the drive-thru guy forgot to give me a napkin. I didn't enjoy my donut quite so much…and I started thinking: Breast cancer is a lot like a jelly donut. The breast *(okay, you had fair warning this book is about bras, boobs, and biopsies)* when healthy, can nourish a new baby with mother's warm milk. The normal cells milk duct contains something wonderful that only a mother can provide. However, when the milk duct becomes filled with invasive ductal cancer cells that leak into the breast, it can be a mess. If it spreads further, lymph nodes can be affected, which terrifies me. A jelly donut, with just the right amount of jelly *(and a napkin)* can be heavenly. But a jelly donut filled with too much jelly *(and no napkin)* can be a mess. The jelly drips down your chin, and if it spreads further, your nice clean white shirt can be ruined. It makes your hands messy, and you feel the sugary grit under your fingernails. Of course this makes us all stop and think about what we do when our hands are donut-messy. We can lick our fingers *(when no one is looking)*, we can use a hand wipe, or we can wash our hands. We all know which option is best, *(and no, not licking our fingers)*. Washing our hands gets rid of the mess.

I can't wait to wash my hands of this horrible disease called cancer. Tomorrow begins the first step. Surgery at 9:45 a.m. Pray no lymph nodes.

The wisdom in this story: I'm having donuts for dinner.

Ready to Fight

Tuesday, October 27

Today's the day.
I'm ready to fight.
One jelly donut at a time.

The wisdom in this story: I'm feeling your prayers. Please pray for clear lymph nodes.

Post-Surgery

Tuesday, October 27

LYMPH NODES CLEAR!!!!!!!
Feeling your prayers.
Waiting for clean margins result.
Please keep praying.
Off to bed with pain meds.

The wisdom in this story: Not impressed with pain meds.

Just Being Mom

Friday, October 30

It is hard for me to accept the many kindnesses of others. On the giving and providing side, I have made many meals throughout the years for others. Sometimes I made beautiful meals for others while my own family was eating boxed macaroni and cheese. I knew how to be a giver, I had learned that from my mom, who always put others first. Yet to receive, especially to *ask* and receive, is very difficult for me. I told everyone we didn't need anything, to which one dear friend replied, "I know, but sometimes you just have to let your friends take care of you. It's what we want to do." Having been on the giving side, I could understand that. Even before surgery, my friends began delivering meals. To be honest, I felt a little guilty. I'm not a very good patient, *(it's hard to keep me down)*. Sometimes a friend delivers a meal and I'm not even home. They tell me that is why they are delivering meals... so I can focus on fighting the cancer and just being Mom. There may come a day when I will have to miss things my kids do, but for now I still have a choice. If I can be there, I will—ice pack, stitches, pain meds, and all. It's been a few rough days. Yet due to the kindness of others who have prepared meals for us and made sure my meds are refilled for the weekend, I can focus on recovering and being just Mom. People have rearranged their lives so that I can live mine. I'm at the football game. It was an uncomfortable ride to State College. Feeling blessed, emotions intact, and then I look down and I see it. My oldest daughter has replaced her red cheer bow with a pink one. I am here, and she knows it.

The wisdom in this story: The cheerleaders need more pink cheer bows.

The Stop Sign

Monday, November 2

As a child, I was tiny — very tiny — and I was never an athlete. I was a "self-proclaimed" wimp. My sister was strong — very strong. She and the neighbor kids once thought it might be funny to tie me to the stop sign with a jump rope. Today, that would be called bullying, involving parents, counselors, and behavior plans, but back then it was just a bump in the road of life on Deerfield Avenue. They didn't leave me there very long, just long enough for me to yell, scream, and feel sorry for myself. I wasn't able to free myself, and they returned a short time later to untie me and be on their way. No apologies, but they never did it again, which made me feel certain that an adult had noticed my helplessness. Years later, my sister couldn't even recall the stop sign incident. The bumps are bigger in life's road now. I'm still a self-proclaimed wimp, but my sister's words from the start of my cancer diagnosis were *"take it one day at a time."* Her words are what make me feel strong. Today was a hard day. I was expecting good news in the pathology report, expecting clean margins from surgery. It wasn't good. Two margins look questionable. They won't share much over the phone. They scheduled me to meet with the surgeon on Wednesday morning. We will talk options in treatment plans and possible surgery to remove more layers. I want to talk about removing everything. The waiting is the hardest part of all of this...I feel tied to the stop sign...just long enough for me to yell, scream, and feel sorry for myself. Then, I hide the helplessness. I pick up and move on, ready to face whatever challenge may be next.

The wisdom in this story: God, you are the one who notices my helplessness. Be with me, and untie the burdens of worry.

Faith, Fear, and Being Brave

Wednesday, November 4

Weeks ago, as I wrote the header for my journal, I wrote "*Let your faith be bigger than your fear,*" *(unknown).* Those were the words that were going to help me get through all of this cancer stuff...but somehow, they were words too quickly forgotten. On what people so affectionately call a cancer journey, it's more than a little easy to feel scared. I feel proud of all that I have already endured, yet scared of all that is yet to come. As you know, my surgery was last week. I cried. Before they even took me into the operating room, I cried. I heard the words, "we'll give you something to make the tears go away, and have you move yourself onto the table." Then it was over—home to heal, and then ready for a plan, a treatment plan. One more hospital bracelet to add to my collection, and a bottle of pills that would make me more restless than tired, yet helped to keep the pain minimal. Visitors, meals, and flowers to make my days brighter, and before I knew it, almost one week had passed. But, then the phone call. "*Margins not clear, the doctor would like to meet with you.*" I didn't shower, I didn't leave the couch, I cried more tears that day than I have throughout this whole ordeal. It was a dozen jelly donuts kind of day. *(Thank goodness there were no donuts in the house!)* But yesterday was a new day. A friend got me out of the house *(hooray!)* and took me to lunch. It was such a treat. We talked about raising teenagers and it felt good to not think about myself. She carefully escorted me to and from the car, and apologized for every bump or curve in the road we traveled. It was so good to get out of the house. I greeted this morning with that same enthusiasm, even though I was on my way to meet with the doctor yet again. We were told she was behind schedule, meeting with a newly diagnosed patient. I felt the tears coming—not for me, not for the wait time, but for the woman in the other room hearing what no woman ever wants to hear. As we waited, the tears came and went. Medical facilities are ugly and boring. They have horrible tissues. The best way I can describe the doctor's entrance to the room was *like a breath of fresh air.* She was calm and patient, caring and reassuring. She shared all that is good *(Stage 1, tumor under 2cm, clear lymph nodes)* and carefully addressed the not so good *(margins not clean).* She explained that I could proceed with treatment, but a more cautious route would be to remove more cancer cells around where the tumor had once been before proceeding. I opted for the second surgery. It seemed like an easy decision. I felt a strong sense of peace, and remembered all who have been praying for me. I felt my faith grow bigger than my fear. I also embraced a new quote I read recently, *"It's okay to be scared. Being scared means you're about to do something really, really brave,"* *(Mandy Hale).* On Tuesday, I will do something really, really brave. I will march back into that hospital wearing my own pink socks *(hospital socks aren't any prettier than MRI socks),* and fight once again. God's got this!

The wisdom in this story: "No matter how you feel, get up, dress up, show up, and never give up," (Regina Brett).

Every Day is a Gift

Thursday, November 5

We are taught not to question God, that every life has a plan, but, sometimes I can't help but wonder. When my mother passed away, it was a quiet, family time. Yet, there were so many at her funeral. The presence of people from my childhood days were a comfort to me. I remember asking people I hadn't seen for years, "How did you know?" Time and time again, they told me they had seen her obituary. The obituaries. When I was a kid, it was the section of the paper that came just before the classified ads; the 110's, a column where puppies were for sale, the page I begged my mother to read with me. *(Yes, I got the puppy!)*. As an adult, that was a page I tried to ignore. I couldn't possibly know anyone *old enough* to die. It wasn't until after my mother's passing at age 66, which everyone solemnly said was "too young," that I started to read the pages each day. Initially, I would scan the names for any that looked familiar, and in time would read the ones that I was oddly drawn to read. These were people. Lives. Busy people with families and loved ones. I prayed for those families. I knew the hurt they were feeling. Today, as I rest and prepare for my next surgery, I'm feeling good. I put some brownies in the oven for a sweet girl I know, and sat down to look at the paper. The obituaries. I first noticed a photograph of a beautiful young woman with the telltale short haircut. Her name was Faith*, age 41. Survived by her adoring husband, mother of four, loved life. In the obituary, her family extended their gratitude to her doctors, nurses, and medical staff who watched over her during her three-and-a-half year battle with *breast cancer*. Directly below the obituary of this woman who was too young to die, was that of another woman named Katherine*. She was 103. The obituary was brief. One hundred three. And then I wondered. Why does 41 even happen, when others can live to be 103? As an educator, it would be simply unacceptable for one student to earn a score of 41, while another student would score a 103. In college, they called it grading on a curve. I loved the curve. I was deep in reflection, wondering about God's curve, and life in general. My cell phone buzzed. I received a text from a dear friend who is fighting her own fight. While she has her own struggles, she never stops thinking about me. The text read:

"Good morning sunshine!
What a beautiful day God
has given us to enjoy.
Hope you are doing well!
Love you!"

And then I realized. It isn't about the number. It isn't about questioning. It is simply about making the best of what we are given, and moving forward. My brother-in-law is an athlete. His endurance and dedication to being fit came as he started realizing the effects of aging. No cholesterol and blood pressure medications for him—he was taking control of his life. He posts regularly about training for his many races and triathlons. He ends most posts with the message, "Every day is a gift, now get out there and enjoy this beautiful day." Every day IS a gift—a beautiful day God has given us to enjoy. I am doing well. I am loved by many. My cancer is curable. I will be a survivor. I think about the dear lady who lived until she was 103. I'm thinking that perhaps even she wanted just a little more time.

The wisdom in this story: I will fight this cancer and win, but I will NEVER train for a triathlon. I like jelly donuts more than jogging.

(*names have been changed)

Surely the Presence

Monday, November 9

I love church. I would love to say that my family attends regularly; but in reality, sometimes work, sports, and even need for sleep interferes with our regular attendance. I know it is an excuse, that plenty of other families with busy schedules tell coaches that church is mandatory, and even doze in the pews a bit so as to not miss a week. I love the calm that fills my days when I start my week with church; but, we show up when we can be there 100%--focused, attentive, and ready to deeply reflect on the message *(well, except for my oldest and youngest who seem to think that church is the time they try to make each other laugh – making faces, pinching, and even the occasional kicking. You would think the 19-year-old would know better, but sometimes he is the instigator).* Anyway, when I'm not there every week, I tend to notice changes. I don't *do* change. I am a routine person. For years I've told my children that church ends right after the offering. So when the offering is moved to before the sermon, even I find it a little difficult to accept that we have awhile to go yet. But I've adjusted. What I do miss is the routine opening with one of my most favorite hymns. Perhaps they still sing it often, *(remember, I'm not there every week)*, but if I recall correctly, *(when my attendance was more regular)* it used to be every week.

Surely the presence of the Lord is in this place.
I can feel His mighty power and His grace.
I can hear the brush of angel's wings,
I see glory on each face.
Surely the presence of the Lord is in this place.
(Lanny Wolfe)

So yesterday at church....they didn't sing it. Yet, it was a song God wanted me to hear, and I had that song in my head all day long. Of course, I started thinking. The presence of the Lord isn't just within the walls of the church. The presence of the Lord is with me always. Throughout this cancer journey I have felt His mighty power and His grace. I have heard the brush of angel's wings with each dear person who has reached out to me, *(especially the nun at the hospital who prayed with me right before my last surgery)*. I see glory on each face, as somehow this awful disease has made me much more aware of the joyfulness in our lives. Yes, surely, the presence of the Lord is with me — *every single day*. Everyone tells me I look wonderful and have a great attitude. A little surgery here and there can't knock me down, *(and praying that chemo and radiation won't either)*, but truly the only way that I can explain my attitude is that I feel your prayers. I feel what I can only describe as a strange sense of calm. It has to be a calm that comes with the presence of the Lord. *(I'm not sure where that presence is on my jelly donut days, but thankfully the jelly donut days have been few. I guess even the Lord feels we need a few jelly donut days)*. So please, dear friends, keep praying. I have another surgery tomorrow. Again, I am terrified. I still hate hospitals. I still hate the ugly socks. I dread the gowns. When they put on my surgical cap last time they told me it was my party hat. I didn't laugh. I am full of anxiety, because that is just the way I am. Yet, I am also feeling the presence of the Lord. Please pray for wisdom for my doctors, and peace and healing for me. This is just another little bump in the road.

The wisdom in this story: I feel your prayers.

For Better or Worse

Tuesday, November 10

I met my husband 29½ years ago. We have been married 22½ years. *Yes, it took us awhile to be sure.* Our vows were traditional. For better or worse. I'm an incredibly independent woman — farm wives need to be. With unpredictable work schedules for my husband, sometimes he was there, sometimes he was not, and it never stopped me from doing as I pleased and taking the kids on adventures. When he was along, it was an extra added bonus, but I never really needed to rely on him. To care for the kids, yes, but not to take care of me. Fast forward to breast cancer. I married a good man. I need him. He is there. He has been with me for every single appointment, every beverage refill, soup warming, and pain pill delivery. For 10 days, I've worn what they call a binding — *the furthest thing from a Victoria's Secret bra you can imagine.* Picture a 70's tube top only much, much wider and sterile, surgical white in color. It's velcro, and I cannot fasten it by myself. He is so very patient. Sometimes he gets it too loose, sometimes too tight, and sometimes mistakenly taps the velcro quite hard right over my tender incision. I don't complain. Believe it or not, breast and lymph nodes incisions can even interfere with putting on one's own socks. I'm a flip-flop girl, so it has been fine...but today, it was time to put on my pink socks for surgery #2. He put on my socks. *I felt like a three-year-old.* Cancer sucks. I asked him if this is what for better or worse means. He laughed. I sure love that man. I told him I don't think we've seen the worst yet. He just smiled his calm, sweet smile, and off we went — back to the hospital. My nurse was a parent whose children went to school with mine. She was wonderful. I'm beginning to think God hand picks everyone that I meet on this journey. My IV Team (*yep, I'm a tricky patient with lousy veins*) couldn't have been more kind as

I winced a little. My anesthesiologist, and surgery nurses were the same ones I had two weeks ago. Before they put me to sleep I had an opportunity to tell them that I wasn't happy to be back there again. They laughed. I wore the ugly party hat. The nurses in the recovery room were wonderful. I needed four warm blankets this time, and each time I asked, they never complained. I had trouble staying awake, and I don't remember their names. Someone even brought me crackers with my apple juice this time. *I think my return visit has earned me VIP status.* While waiting to be discharged, my son sent me a text with a photo of a beautiful cake. One of my dearest friends moved to Florida, but remembered the name of the best local bakery and had a cake delivered. I told my husband we have good people in our lives. It was the first time today that I felt my eyes fill with tears. I told him that I knew we had good people in our lives, that I didn't need this awful disease to remind me. But it has reminded me — tenfold. The incredible gestures of so many have warmed my heart. I feel so very loved. Cancer does that. It also makes us stop to realize that we don't say "I love you" often enough. The surgery went as planned, the doctor removed 1 cm more, *(goodbye, cancer)* and it too, will now be tested. Tomorrow I meet with the medical oncologist and on Friday I meet with the radiation oncologist. I am continually reminded of my sister's words....one day at a time. I'm doing well, more sore than I expected, but ready for what comes next. The note that came with my friend's cake said "You deserve more than just a jelly donut." It made me laugh. What started as my first-ever major cancer pity party has turned into a wonderful joke between friends. The cake was heavenly...a white chocolate raspberry torte...*layers of white cake filled with raspberry filling, iced with white chocolate mousse, and garnished with white chocolate, shavings, and raspberry jelly.* When this journey is over and they call me a Survivor, I'm having a party. You are all invited. I have a lot of good people in my life. I will still be an incredibly independent woman, but I'll have a proud man standing by my side. He will be serving jelly donuts. The cake, you ask—I will be delivering one of those to Florida.

The wisdom in this story: I married a good man, and we are blessed to have such good people in our lives. I love each and every one of you.

Do the Math

Thursday, November 12

I had my appointment with the medical oncologist yesterday. I had hoped to see the same doctor who treated my mother 16 years ago, but she was on vacation. I met with another wonderful doctor. The new patient paperwork stated that one should allow approximately two hours for the first visit. *I wondered how the first visit could possibly take two hours.* I was there two hours. The visit started with more bloodwork. I asked what it was for, as I've had several sticks over the course of the past several weeks. They told me they needed all of my blood counts before the start of any treatment. It reminded me of my job as an educator. Benchmark assessments — kids cry, teachers complain, and yet we end up with a tidy little column of numbers that really does accurately help us plan a course of learning for our students. So three needle sticks *(yep, they couldn't find a good vein)* and four vials of blood later, they had more of what they needed to accurately plan a course of treatment for me. I listened to the doctor talk, for a long time. She was thorough, very knowledgeable, and careful to be sure that I understood everything she was saying. Again, I was reminded of being on the teacher side of the desk. How often we are guilty of throwing around teacher terminology and acronyms without stopping to think that the parent must understand. Well, this doctor was good at what she does. She made sure the patient understood. Everything. She had many good things to say. The tumor, while not "teeny," *(I smiled to hear her use that word),* wasn't huge. It measured 1.5 cm. As I had learned previously, under 2 cm is easier to treat. Praise God. Two lymph nodes were negative for cancer, which placed this cancer in Stage 1 category. They give the tumor a grade, based on how abnormal the cells and tumor tissue look under a microscope. It is an indicator of how quickly a tumor is likely to grow and spread. A 1 looks pretty good, 3 is faster growing and spreads quickly. Mine is a 2. My hormone receptors were estrogen + and progesterone +, which indicates less chance of spreading into the body. I was also HER-2 negative, which she said is good. She said with the re-excision surgery I had on Tuesday, the cancer could be gone. I could be *cured*, BUT then she also said that there could be a 50% chance of remaining cancer cells. There is a test...the Oncotype-DX test. In my mind, it is the final exam of the semester. While most other factors appear negative for chemo need, this test is the big one, the deciding factor. With a low or middle score, chemo may not be beneficial. If the score is high, then chemo. My tumor is in sunny California being tested, and I won't have a result until next week. I will get a phone call first, then follow up with the medical oncologist on November 24th, and finally, I will have a plan. In the meantime, I am reminded how as educators we sandwich our words to parents. You know, it's the positive comment, a quick concern in the middle, and then ending on another happy note. *(i.e. Johnny is an excellent reader. He has difficulty staying focused. Johnny is a kind friend to others)*. Aww... Johnny is awesome. There's just that little problem in the middle. I'm praying that with all of the factors stacked up, my Oncotype-DX isn't that little problem in the middle. Because the rest truly looks good:

Under 2 cm
2 lymph nodes negative
Stage 1
Grade 2 (grade 1 would have been better, but it's not a 3)
estrogen +
progesterone +
HER2 –
re-excision surgery

That's a whole lot of happy all in one tidy little column.

So now, I wait—*again*. But, back to the numbers—I never felt like just a number yesterday. I was a patient, seated across the desk from a doctor who cared—a doctor who truly cared. She asked for my mother's name. She wondered if she knew my mom. This doctor started with the group in January 2001. My mom started with Hospice in February 2001. She pulled up my mother's chart anyway. She told me that for many years, they numbered their patients. My mother was patient number 12,939. Sixteen years later, they have now seen over 80,000 patients. Do the math. That's a whole lot of cancer, a whole lot of patients, and yet a doctor who was more than willing to spend two hours talking to me about my cancer and treatment options. I continue to pray that I don't need chemo. But whatever comes next, I'm ready to fight. I learned from the best...patient number 12,939...my mom.

The wisdom in this story: Always focus on the positive.

Be the Boss

Sunday, November 15

There is no doubt about it, I like to be the boss — of everything. I am an in-charge kind of person. I like things my way. My mother always told me that I would have been an incredible attorney. I like to win. There is nothing quite like a cancer diagnosis to remind you that you are not always the boss. You are not always in charge. You don't always get things your way. *But, fight like hell, and you can win.* I met with the radiation oncologist on Friday. While the medical oncologist spent two hours explaining absolutely everything to us, this particular doctor spent probably about two minutes. He rattled off the statistics of patients who receive radiation treatment, and told me that I will receive a total of 33 treatments/every day for 7 weeks. With radiation, there will only be a 5% chance of recurrence. I'll be swollen, tender, and have red, dry, flaky, itchy skin. "And that's about it. Any questions? The nurse will be in to see you shortly." My husband and I both sat there with what I can only describe as the deer in headlights look. When the nurse walked in the door, I couldn't help but comment, "he was so fast, so *very* fast." While I didn't really have questions, I have found throughout this journey it is the fear of the unknown that causes me anxiety. The nurse offered to explain things now, when I come for simulation, or both times. She assured me that she had time to talk with us, and I gratefully accepted. She couldn't have been more kind. She explained every single step. She showed me the equipment. She gave me a packet of information and a list of products that I can safely use to treat my skin during radiation. I went from feeling helpless and overwhelmed, to feeling a part of the plan. Even if that plan meant simply adding a certain kind of soap to my shopping list, I was again in charge. I was the boss. I thought about my interactions with both doctors. One, two hours...the other, two minutes . They are both highly respected experts in their field, but only one chose to join my pity party. Only one offered the true compassion that I so desperately seem to need. Thank heavens for the nurse that spent more time with me. While each and every individual I meet along this path is part of my healing, it's really all up to me. Attitude is everything. A long time ago, I wrote "I choose happy." Some days that is hard. The recovery from this second surgery is not as fast as I had anticipated. On Friday, I told my husband I felt like crap. He gently reminded me that I was only three days out from surgery. I am not a patient kind of patient. I need to be the boss. Of everything. I need to be in charge. I like things my way. I'm ready to fight like hell and win — as soon as I get my energy back. Today, I still feel crappy. And a little sad. Not quite jelly donut status, but almost. Life is good. The sun is shining. My youngest daughter tells me it is 39 days, 11 hours, 32 minutes until Christmas. We have shopping to do. A mild bar soap is on my list — that sweet smell of childhood that reminds me of my mother, who knew that I like to win.

The wisdom in this story: I am the boss of this cancer.

Not a Patient Patient

Wednesday, November 18

Today, I put on my 11th gown *(as in medical gown, not fancy gown)* since this journey has started. But who's counting? I'm counting. Yes. Eleven. All ugly. Some too big, some too small. Some with an effort to match the ugly examining rooms, and none with any respect for those of us who are even slightly modest. Okay, I'm *very* modest. It's been a rough few days. I developed a low-grade fever over the weekend and fell into a miserable *slump (albeit my slump-i-ness did not prevent me from attending a football game, a cheerleading competition, and a dairy meeting)*. On Monday night, I had the pity party of all pity parties *(sans jelly donuts)*. Most of my pity parties are in my alone times, in the quiet stillness of an empty house. This one erupted from nowhere, me simply rambling for at least 10 minutes to a bewildered-looking husband about how unfair all of this is, and how *(yes, woe is me)* I do not *deserve* this. I told him I think I'm a good person and I always put others first. Through tears I shouted, "and I'm not even mean." After I said those words, I realized how silly and selfish I must have sounded. Even mean people don't deserve cancer...no one *deserves* cancer. My little pity party *(more like temper tantrum meltdown)* has bothered me. I don't usually like *that side* of me to emerge. I chalked it all up to anxiety with awaiting results for my OncotypeDX *(test on the tumor to determine need for chemo)*. I thought I would get that result today, at my post-op appointment. As my day started, I was irritable at best. Slow to shower, reluctant to handle some school issues related to my absence, and just generally grumpy. As my husband and I got on the elevator at the surgeon's office *(for what felt like the hundredth time)*, I pointed out to him the ugliness of the bulletin board and the disarray of papers randomly tacked on it. Am I really that OCD...or am I just *"not a patient patient."* One of my greatest complaints throughout this ordeal, *(yep,*

50

my mood today prevents me from calling it a "journey") has been in the small stuff. The awkward gowns, the horrible socks, the ugly examining rooms, and yes...even the bulletin board. I did notice that the bulletin board had one pink crystal tack, but even that didn't make me smile. The doctor's office did not have my test result yet. More waiting. Maybe Friday. Even the lovely nurse who delivered chocolate to everyone in the waiting room didn't make me smile. *Okay, I smiled, but only long enough for the snack size chocolate to satisfy my soul.* When the doctor asked me how I was doing, I was honest. I told her I wasn't recovering as quickly as I had hoped. I told her my husband reminded me it has only been a week since surgery. She smiled, and gave him a knowing look. I told her I'm not a patient patient. She told me that sometimes low grade fevers after surgery indicate not enough deep breaths. Perhaps I needed to get up and move around a bit more. I didn't tell her about the football game, the cheer competition, and the princess meeting. In my own mind, I wondered if low grade fevers after surgery can also indicate doing too much. But I thought that should be my little secret. Once again, the doctor's calm reassuring manner helped me to relax. Once again, I remembered my sister's words to take everything one day at a time. I didn't notice the bulletin board on the elevator ride down. As I walked out into the breezy fall day, I was ready to search online, but this time not about cancer. I wanted the dictionary definition of patient. And this is what I learned:

pa*tient
/paSHent/

noun
a person receiving or registered to receive medical treatment. A sick person.

adjective
to be able to accept or tolerate delays, problems, or suffering
without becoming annoyed or anxious.

In summary, I have been a patient since September 24th. I
have received, and will be registered to receive medical
treatment. I am a sick person. I am a patient. However, I have
NOT been able to accept or tolerate delays *(in receiving test
results)*, problems *(not one surgery but two)*, and suffering *(yep, I
still hurt)* without becoming annoyed *(about the small things,
like the socks)* or anxious *(about the waiting)*. So, it is best to say
"I am not a patient patient."

But, I am not mean. Sometimes people are mean. A lady in the
waiting room wanted to complain to me about the wait. I told
her that sometimes I'm the reason the doctor is behind
schedule, so I try to be compassionate if others need a little
extra time to accept a cancer diagnosis. She didn't accept the
chocolate from the cheerful nurse. *Who doesn't accept the
chocolate?* She told me she didn't live close by, that they should
have called her to tell her that they were behind schedule. I
did wonder why technology hasn't allowed for this *(after all,
the white board that announced the doctor's one hour behind
schedule and was then erased to announce two hours behind
schedule does seem a little 1980s)*. My favorite steakhouse can
text me when my table is ready, so surely there is some way
the medical field could accommodate those who have less
time to wait. So I guess sometimes, when I have to wait for
others, I can be patient. And above all else, I try to be a good
person and put others first. I try not to be mean. But even the
mean lady in the waiting room...she doesn't deserve cancer.

I came home to the loveliest package of chocolates in my
mailbox *(and a note about a jelly donut)* from the parent of a
student I had 25 years ago. There's something special about
people who choose to stay in your life that long. The

seasonal candy is a chocolate assortment of snowflakes. I'm ready for snow. I'm ready for the next step in my journey, whatever it may be. Chocolate does sweeten everything. I'd like to eat the whole bag, but I just might save it, I know a nurse who may need to replenish her stash.

The wisdom in this story: Cancer books contain "fluff" — the feel good stories everyone wants to hear. My stories are real. Raw emotion, temper tantrums and all — the truth about cancer. The truth about every ugly gown, sock, examining room, and bulletin board. And if you have read yet another one of my very long narratives, may God bless you. You are a good person. You put others first. You put me first. And if you are mean...I have chocolate...and I share.

I Need Chemo

Tuesday, November 24

Well, exactly two months ago today, I had a mammogram. The result of said mammogram has been a whirlwind of emotion, a whole lot of waiting, and whole lot of uncertainty. During this time, I've learned to appreciate the beauty in each day, and the cleansing tears that sometimes come in the quiet times. What has been most frustrating to Type A Personality Me *(okay OCD, too)* has been the lack of a plan. I'm a calendar person. A planner. An organizer. I like to be in charge. The boss. As of today, I have a plan *(and yes, I am the boss of this cancer)*. I need chemo. I. NEED. CHEMO. *(I know the punctuation is out of place, but those are just the words "sinking in...")* While I sound strong, I am heartbroken. There is not room on my calendar for it. It's not part of *MY* plan. And yet it has to be. Things on the calendar must be rearranged and chemo (every 21 days for four treatments) will be a part of my plan. My new normal, followed by seven weeks/33 rounds of radiation. I'm optimistic. Is there really another choice? The donut shop simply doesn't have enough jelly donuts in stock to handle this most recent blow. The best IV nurse in the oncologist's office checked my veins, and apparently the hospital IV team's definition of *tricky* suits me perfectly. They won't be able to run the chemo through my veins. I will need a port. My dear friend once had a port. She loved her port. I begged my mother to get a port to escape her many needle pricks, sores, and bruises. She refused. I think she was proud of her battle scars. I wanted to refuse the port, but it wasn't really a choice. So, (hopefully next week) I will return to the hospital for a port. Once I have the port, chemo can be started immediately. I am hoping for Thursdays. A teacher I met at the surgeon's office told me she "went for chemo treatments on Thursday, dragged her ass *(her words, not mine)* into school on Friday, and rested over the weekend." She was back to school by Monday. I am praying to be so fortunate. I will get anti- nausea meds, followed by two chemo drugs, and will be at the oncologist's office for about three hours. The next day, I will return for an injection that should help rebuild my white blood cells. I will lose my hair. I. WILL. LOSE. MY. HAIR. *(Again, words sinking in...).* I asked about hair at my first oncology appointment. I don't care about my hair for me, or for the opinions of my friends and family. I do care about my hair for my first graders and all of the kids in my school. They will know. The word cancer will enter some of their vocabularies. And it could be awful. But I won't let it be awful. Yet, they will see me without hair. I will not get a wig. I decided this a long time ago. At one of my first visits to the breast surgeon, I browsed the booklet of wigs. They all looked perfect. My hair never looks perfect. I'm more of a windblown type of gal — wash and wear. I would look silly in a real wig. So, my plan is to look even sillier. I'll wear hats and scarves, but the highlight of my days will be the occasions when I make my six-year-olds laugh with colorful wigs. I'm planning a school-themed polar bear purple for winter, hot pink for Valentine's Day, and even green in March to show off my Irish heritage. I won't wear a wig every day — hot and itchy are the words that come to mind. But as my sister says...one day at a time. I doubt she realizes it, but her words are what keep me going...*every single day.* I think of what others have said to me:

"God never gives us more than we can handle," *(I'm not so sure.)*

"You are the strongest person I know." *(Ahem, do you KNOW how many jelly donuts I have eaten?").*

"It could be so much worse." *(This one I agree with...there are children with cancer.)*

"Everything happens for a reason." *(more on this later...)*

"Your family will be so close after this experience." *(We were already extremely close.)*

"You can handle anything." *(I'm not so sure...)*

"It's all part of God's plan." *(This one I agree with, too...but it's still hard to accept.)*

"You have so many people who care about you." *(Absolutely, and I feel very blessed.)*

But the best thing ever, came in the form of a card from a retired teacher friend who has fought her own battle. The card says,

"Please let me
be the first
to punch
the next person
who tells you
everything happens
for a reason."
(Empathy Cards by Emily McDowell)

Beautiful, heartfelt cards and letters from friends and loved ones flood my mailbox daily. That card will always be my favorite. Even if everything truly does happen for a reason, *cancer sucks.* There is no nice way to say it. I am heartbroken. But finally, after two full months of waiting, I have a plan. The steps to follow will lead me to being cured. A survivor. Those are the best words ever. Just two days before my diagnosis, our local newspaper ran an article for National Breast Cancer Awareness Month. The article featured a cancer patient who is a teacher in a local school. She has given me permission to share. My favorite interview question follows:

Q: "How can people be truly helpful to a woman being treated for breast cancer?"

A: "No sad eyes. I hated going places and people would look at me with sad eyes. It was always the adults that would do that, and I understand, but it made it hard."

She also said that her loved ones rallied to help her keep her normal life as she battled cancer. She relies on her husband, son, and her students to cheer her on in what she calls the fight of her life.

I'm preparing for the fight of my life. My loved ones will rally to help me keep my normal life as I battle cancer. I will rely on my husband, children, and my students to cheer me on in this fight.

The wisdom in this story: No sad eyes. I choose happy. And sometimes, happy means colorful wigs.

A Snoopy Sign

Tuesday, November 24

Two months ago, "*Get Peanutized*" was all over the internet. I had always loved Charles Shultz, but had an even greater affection for him when I learned that *(just like my mother)* he had colon cancer. He died a year and a half before my mom. On September 23, I tried to make myself into a Peanuts character. I don't usually participate in these online games, but this was too tempting not to try. I tried several outfits — my high school colors of red, white, and black; my college sorority colors of pink and green; and purple, the color of the school where I teach. I tried various hairstyles and found a great pink bracelet. When I clicked post your image, it posted me — totally bald. My daughter laughed. My tone grew serious. "It's not funny. It's like a sick person, someone with cancer." Now, I'm not tech savvy, but with my daughter's assistance, we tried again. Different hair. Post. Bald. Again. I gave up on being a Peanuts character. The next day, I went for my mammogram. You know the rest of the story. Two months have passed. I start chemo very soon. The oncologist said that I will most definitely lose my hair. For many, many years I have asked God to send me some sort of sign that mom is with me. I know this sounds silly, but I think she and Charles Shultz sent one.

The wisdom in this story: I can only hope I'll be as beautiful as the Peanuts character I created.

At This Very Moment

Friday, November 27

I truly try to not wear my heart on my sleeve. I try to keep my pity parties to my alone times *(with a jelly donut, of course)*. I try to be my happy self as much as humanly possible for a cancer patient. But quite frankly, my world has crashed. I've missed a month of work, and I'm about to tell an adorable class of first graders why I'll lose my hair. I face the reality that the mom who always attends everything in which her children participate, might have to miss some things. And in case you have forgotten, I'm the person who is terrified of most anything medical. I'm a self-proclaimed wimp, and the tests, needle pricks, surgeries, and long-awaited phone calls with disappointing test results haven't helped. That fear of the unknown will remain a part of my world throughout the months of treatments that lie ahead, and in the wait for the five-year-word, survivor. I'll lose my hair, but what else? Will my illness during winter months exacerbate the usual effects of spending hours indoors with first grade germs? Will my body be able to handle the harsher chemo drugs every 21 days, or will we need to change course and stretch things out to lessen side effects, which will in turn make this whole process longer? Will the nausea meds help, or will I be vomiting? Will I need anti-diarrheal for diarrhea or stool softener for constipation...they told me either could be possible? Will I get the dreaded mouth sores that made my mother feel so miserable? Will I have any lasting side-effects from the estrogen receptor drug that I'll need to take for five years? Will my insurance cover all of my medical bills? Will my loss of pay with missed work prevent me from even being able to pay my regular household bills? Will I cry? So sometimes, in my weaker moments, I wear my heart on my sleeve. I openly admit that I am struggling. I inadvertently try to pull others into my pity party. Some listen kindly as I ramble. Others hold my hand in silence. Some tell me that they're going to buy me more jelly donuts. But there are some people who feel the need to tell me that there are others who have things so much worse. I'm not sure why they feel the need to share — perhaps when one mentions the word cancer they don't truly know what to say, so they tell you about someone they know who has cancer. Perhaps it's to silence my pity party that feels so awkward when I'm usually fairly upbeat and pleasant to be around. But in my mind, it somehow seems that they are trying to minimize my situation and I feel worse. Sometimes these are the same people who criticized my original surgery decision of lumpectomy vs. mastectomy *(something that was truly discussed at great lengths with a surgeon I respect and trust)*. I am very aware that things are much, much worse in the world. I was diagnosed Stage 1. Curable. It will be a long road, but I will be cured. Others are not so fortunate. As I mentioned in a recent story, there are families who are dealing with childhood cancers. There are heart attacks, car accidents, even suicides that leave families devastated. So, in the grand scheme of the world, an aggressive Invasive Ductal Carcinoma Stage 1, really isn't such a terrible thing. I know that things are much, much worse in the world. *But in MY world, at this very moment, it is awful.*

A few favorite quotes come to mind:

"Don't judge a man until you've walked a mile in his shoes." *(American Proverb)*

"Before you start to judge me, step into my shoes and walk the life I'm living. If you get as far as I am, just maybe you will see how strong I really am." *(unknown)*

"Judging a person does not define who they are...it defines who you are." *(unknown)*

"Don't judge my path if you haven't walked my journey."
(unknown)

To say that I'm a little sensitive these days is a bit of an understatement. The tears sometimes come out of nowhere. Perhaps no one is actually judging my decisions, my pity parties, or my self-sorrow. Maybe, to me it just seems that way. Maybe I'm secretly a bit envious of those whose biggest challenge of the day is deciding which outfit to wear or what to make for dinner. That was me once. But when cancer *(even Stage 1)* enters your world, everything seems to change. This, too shall pass. I am reminded of what my youngest daughter's doctor said about her bad ankle sprain. The recovery will be longer than it is short. My cancer journey will be the same — longer than it is short. In the meantime, bless you for being patient with my sadness.

The wisdom in this story: Everyone you meet is fighting a battle you know nothing about. Be kind. Always. (unknown)

On Time for Church

Sunday, November 29

Many years ago, our early church service started at 8:45 a.m.
Then, due to parking issues, someone had the brilliant idea to
start the service at 8:15 a.m. Surely no one with small children
in their homes was part of that decision! It was a struggle.
Each Sunday, no matter how hard we tried, we rolled into the
parking lot promptly at 8:25 a.m. We were exactly 10 minutes
late for the service, almost every time. We found solace in the
fact that another family *(also with three children)* arrived with
us at 8:25 a.m. We jokingly said that we were part of our own
8:25 a.m. service. Now, I would be remiss if I did not
recognize one amazing family *(with four children)* who always
managed to be on time. Mom wore beautiful clothes, very
high heels, and never appeared to struggle with the toddler
she juggled on her hip. Her hair was always beautifully styled
and makeup perfect. *I felt like an unmade bed.* My husband and
I often wondered how she did it! Fast forward several years,
and it is still a struggle for our family to get to church on time.
Sometimes it's slow-moving teenagers that delay us, but lately
it has been me. I'm fast in the shower, and do very little with
makeup, but it's the hair. Now it's not beautifully styled, but
it's very thick and takes forever to blow dry. Today, in spite of
my best efforts, Morgan and I arrived at church just as the
prelude was beginning. The sermon was fabulous. The title of
the sermon was GODISNOWHERE, and was listed as such
(all bold capitals, no spaces) in the bulletin. As I read *"God is
Nowhere,"* I thought that perhaps this sermon was written just
for me. I have questioned. I have wondered. I have asked
why. I have even asked where God is along my journey. While
my faith has taught me to know that God is always with me,
that He walks before me, I have still questioned. Pastor told us
to turn and talk with others, to guess what the sermon title
meant. I looked at a very wise, elderly *(but young at heart)*

gentleman beside me who has struggled greatly with health issues. I shrugged my shoulders. I thought the sermon title was odd. He smiled, and very proudly stated *"God is Now Here."* What I read as *"God is Nowhere,"* was now very clearly (with spaces in the right places) *"God is Now Here."* WOW! What a powerful message. The sermon that followed was equally wonderful, and the message touched me deeply. Ironically, my glass-always-full oldest daughter had immediately read it as *"God is Now Here."* Our pastor reminded us that even with our joys, there are sorrows. He reminded us that in our deepest, darkest moments, God is with us. GOD IS NOW HERE. Our Advent prayer brought tears to my eyes.

O God of Hope, we praise you
that into this world of darkness,
you sent your Son to be the
true light illumining everyone.
Help us to see the signs that Christ
is with us, and to bring the light
of His hope into the lives
of those around us. Amen.
(Responsive Calls to Worship)

This day reminded me of some of my early online journal pages. My words were *"I choose happy"* and *"Let your faith be bigger than your fear."* Somehow, within the mix of words surgeries, port, chemo, and radiation I lost sight of the word cure. Somehow my glass started becoming more empty, my world a little darker, my acknowledgement that Christ is with us a little too far from my thoughts. Yet, today I was reminded. Life is good. Even with sorrows, there can be joy. As I think about the chemo to come and the impending loss of my thick, beautiful hair, it saddens me. However, I will choose to focus on the positive. Maybe, just maybe, I will now be on time for church. Then again, I'm not yet an expert at tying the scarves cancer patients wear on their bald heads. So if you want to meet up with me in the parking lot, I'll be the one arriving at 8:25 a.m. About the lady who wore beautiful clothes, very high heels, and never appeared to struggle—her hair is still beautifully styled and makeup perfect. She still wears beautiful clothes and high heels. She arrives on time, even early—and she is my church friend. I look forward to her bright cheerful smiles when our paths cross. She is one of the few faces still familiar to me in a church that has grown and changed throughout the many years we have attended. We have our own personal joke that she sometimes sits in my pew. But most Sundays, my pew is empty. I think she now attends the 10:45 a.m. service. If I can't tie the scarf, I might be joining her for the late service!

The wisdom in this story: Even in our sorrows, there are joys.

They are Six

Wednesday, December 2

It's so good to be back at school again. Yesterday and today have exhausted me, but my absence reminded me that *(even after 26 years of teaching)* I do belong in the classroom. I have enjoyed two wonderful days with my first graders, and a never-ending flow of big kids returning to visit me. *(Apparently, word got out that I've been missing).* The hugs from my first graders seem endless *(and you know just where six-year-olds reach to hug – thank goodness for a compression bra and a bit of padding to cover my still-tender incision!).* There is something so incredibly wonderful about six-year-olds. Like me, their emotions are raw. They get angry. They have tantrums. They say what they think. They have no filter. And then it's all over and we are moving on to something better. In my absence, the substitute teacher struggled with student behaviors. I maintain a very well-managed classroom, and never have to raise my voice. They know I have high expectations and they do not disappoint. I treat them with respect, and they are respectful in return. However when someone new comes along, they're smart enough to test the boundaries a bit, and test they did. I felt sorry for my substitute, and her days were challenging. One student decided that he would stick his tongue out at the substitute teacher — quite obviously not a good choice. And yet, he is charming. I asked this student to explain what happened with the substitute. "I stick-ded my tongue out at her." When I told him that disappointed me deeply, and asked why he would do such a thing, he responded, "I just missed you so much." We talked about some better ways he could have handled missing me, and big tears fell from his eyes. This is hard. This is all hard. I am what they know and love, and different is hard. Under other exciting circumstances like my maternity leaves, I walked out the door and never looked back. I had confidence that any

65

qualified substitute could excel in my absence. My feelings are different this time. I am leaving them for a different reason. While these many appointments and treatments are hard for me, they are also hard for my students. They are six. As the oncologist feels certain I will lose my hair, I felt that it would be best to talk to the students in advance. Initially, I asked my guidance counselor to do it, because I didn't think I could talk without crying. Then I tried to imagine myself sitting off to the side listening while she talked to them, and I didn't like that idea either. So I did what I do best—I wrote a creative lesson plan. I will be absent from school again tomorrow to get a medi-port (and I pray that my students behave for the substitute), but I will be back on Friday. On Friday, my students will learn about the word cancer. I've got my cheering squad (counselor, nurse, principal, and some wonderful support staff) joining me for moral support, and I have invited the parents to attend. I know that may sound odd, but I think I would want to be present if someone was telling my six-year-old about cancer. I will be telling them about the "not-so-good things, the good things, and the BEST things about cancer." When I talked to one of our building aides about my plan, she asked, "what IS good about cancer?" To be honest, I'm not sure. What I do know is that I can do a pretty awesome job convincing first graders just about anything! So here's what they will learn:

I have missed school because I have cancer.

Cancer is something growing in your body that doesn't belong. I had surgery and my doctor took it out.

Doctors don't really know what causes cancer. They work hard every day to find out.

Sometimes people wonder, can you "catch" it?
We will talk about how you can "catch" a cold, pink eye, the flu,

a sore throat, a fever, and even head lice. Yes, head lice. Been there done that. We will talk about how you can NOT "catch" a loose tooth, a bruise, an ear ache, broken bones, or a paper cut. We will talk about how you can NOT "catch" cancer. Whew!

Even though the doctors took my cancer out, I still need some medicines to help make sure the cancer does not come back. That is called treatment.

Sometimes cancer makes people feel sad.

Sometimes things about cancer are not good.
1. *I might be tired.*
2. *I might get sick.*
3. *I will miss some school.*
4. *I will lose my hair.*

In life, with every sad, there is also a happy. (Thanks, Pastor!)

There are good things.
1. *I might be tired, but:*
    Family takes good care of me.
    Friends take good care of me.
2. *I might get sick, but:*
    My cancer doesn't hurt.
    I have amazing doctors.
    Doctors have good medicines.
3. *I will miss some school, but:*
    We have great substitutes.
    I will get better soon.
4. *I will lose my hair, but:*
    Scarves are pretty.
    Wigs can be silly.

I could feel sad and think about the not-so-good-good things, but I choose happy.

We are going to talk about the BEST things about cancer.

1. *I might be tired, but:*
      *You can be my best helpers.
      *Pajama Days are awesome.
      *You can wake me if I snore.
2. *I might get sick, but:*
      *We will be germ chasers.
      *We have the best hand sanitizer.
3. *I will miss school, but:*
      *We love Mrs. (insert substitute's name here).
4. *I will lose my hair, but:*
      *Hat days will be fun.

People need to know about cancer. They need to know that with sad, there is always happy. Teaching people about cancer is called awareness. People use colorful ribbons to show awareness about cancers. The color for breast cancer awareness is pink. Our classroom has its very own pink ribbon. I also put pink ribbons on our calendar to show which days I have cancer treatments.

I shared my story with you because you are a part of my team. Sometimes teams have special wristbands. These pink wristbands say HOPE because we hope that someday there will be no cancer in the world. These pink wristbands say STRENGTH because you help me to be strong as I fight the cancer. These pink wristbands say LOVE because it is always important to tell someone you love them. Sometimes cancer reminds us to say *"I love you."*

Thank you for being a part of my TEAM.

I WILL GET BETTER.

Suffice it to say, this is perhaps the hardest lesson I've ever written. I have pretty pink graphic organizer cards, a scarf and an obnoxiously purple wig to show, the enticing smell of sweet scented hand sanitizers, the promise of a pink wristband, and the anticipation of Pajama Days, Hat Days, and the possibility of seeing their teacher snore. Kids will giggle. Adults will cry. And my story will once again be told. Cancer is awful. However, first graders don't need to know that. I might look a little different, but I am still Mrs. Brymesser — First Grade Teacher. Cancer will not get in the way of our learning. My journey will be longer than it is short, but in the end I will have taught them the life lesson of fighting and being a survivor. Someday when they hear the word cancer again in the life of someone they love, they will not be terrified. They will remember me and know that even a world with cancer can be happy and fun. Being able to stay focused on your inner strength is an important lesson in childhood, and actually in life. As adults, it is our role to cultivate resiliency. We need to cultivate optimism, focus on strengths, and be accepting of change. We need to teach our children to look on the bright side. Life is good.

The wisdom in this story: Sometimes it's okay to get angry, have tantrums, and say what you think. It is even okay to stick your tongue out at cancer, but NEVER, EVER stick your tongue out at the substitute teacher!

The Easy Button

Thursday, December 3

Years ago, an office supply store introduced the *Easy Button*. I promptly put one on my teacher desk for students to press during challenging writing workshops. They are always a bit curious about it during the first marking period *(I don't start formal writing workshop until marking period 2)*, and somehow the anticipation of actually pushing it makes it all the more rewarding when they get to use it. Today, I went back to the hospital for a medi-port procedure *(to eliminate the need for needle sticks and the possibility of chemo burns during treatment with my oh-so-uncooperative veins)*. I expected to be in and out, and jokingly compared it a bit to micro-chipping a dog. The hospital informed me that I should plan on a five-hour hospital stay, as the procedure alone took at least an hour. They said I would receive twilight sedation, and I politely requested that I be more asleep than awake. While some people like to know what the doctors are doing, I'd rather not know. *Wake me when it's over.* While in recovery, they told me that my blood pressure had dropped and my heart rate had increased during the procedure. They told me I wasn't breathing properly, and asked me if I remembered the nurse telling me to take deep breaths of the oxygen they had provided. All of that scared me a bit. I've never been anything less than the happily sedated patient. Perhaps "twilight" isn't the way to go for me. They told me later the troubles were partly due to having received a lot of medication, and also my anxiety. *Anxiety. Who me?* It seemed to take awhile for me to feel fully awake, and my blood pressure was taken every 15 minutes until it seemed satisfactory enough to send me home. So—after a day of bloodwork, IV, another ugly gown, more bright yellow socks, twilight sedation, a medi-port procedure, and a long time for my patient husband to wait, I am home—*home and grumpy.* They said I shouldn't have pain, just a dull ache. I hurt like hell. *(Sorry, no nice way to say it).* But, as I am learning, this too shall pass. With each extra-strength acetaminophen *(I hate acetaminophen, but I hate prescription drugs more)*, my pain will lessen and I will begin to feel normal again. Probably just in time for them to knock me down again with Chemotherapy Treatment #1. However, I know that with my chemo, I won't need any needle sticks. Every blood draw, chemo infusion, medication, and IV fluid will now go in through my medi-port, which I'm choosing to call my easy button. If just one small thing about this whole process is made easier, and that button helps ease my frustrations, today's scary procedure will have been worth it. First graders become quite frustrated with the process of Writing Workshop. They give you what they think is their best, and it's not quite enough. They are sent back to revise, edit, and try again. The easy button helps keep the tears away. They are always proud of the end result. I have become quite frustrated with the process of fighting cancer. The surgery wasn't enough. The second surgery wasn't enough. The chemo won't be enough. Finally, when I finish chemo and radiation *(sometime in April or May)*, I will be done. I will be proud of the end result. I am just hopeful my easy button/port helps keep the tears away along the way.

The wisdom in this story: Sometimes overcoming the struggles in life is all about convincing oneself. Even when we don't agree, the little button reminds us, "That was easy."

The Flat Tire

Friday, December 4

Today, I taught the hardest lesson of my career. I taught my students about cancer. I avoided eye contact with the crying parents, my colleagues, and my oldest daughter, who joined me for moral support, *(and to model the hats, scarves, and wigs – bless her heart!)*. I focused only on my students, and taught the lesson as I teach everything else: with need-to-know information, gentle words, and a touch of humor. My students' eyes were serious and they listened intently; but when appropriate, they giggled loudly. Oh, how I love first grade giggles! When it was their turn to share, one little girl tearfully told us that my story reminded her of her grandmother's dog. Another student told us his father needed surgery because he was in a car accident. As things often go in first grade, that story led to another student's dramatic retelling of his mother's flat tire. *A flat tire.* I tried not to laugh. Everyone describes this cancer journey as a little bump in the road. Some days, I feel like I'm chugging along just fine, and other days my tire is flat. The port is hurting more than I had anticipated, and my anxiety increases daily about the chemo to come next week. But my cancer, like the flat tire, can be fixed. For flat tires, we call a three-lettered automobile association. For my cancer, I count on FFF *(Faith, Family, and Friends)*. Today my tire was feeling flat, but was a good day. My principal liked the lesson. My guidance counselor was surprised I wrote the lesson. Someone else commented that I should publish the lesson. My daughter *(who aspires to be a teacher)* was just thrilled to be in the classroom. As I had hoped, my students learned that while cancer can be sad, there is always a happy. But the best part of today – I didn't cry. With the help of my faith, family, and friends *(and some fabulous first graders)*, I am ready to fight.

The wisdom in this story:

Faith: Seeing light with your heart when all your eyes see is darkness.

Family: God's gift to you, as you are to them.

Friends: Angels who lift us up when our own wings have trouble remembering how to fly.

(unknown)

Really?

Sunday, December 6

Circa 1976, I loved everything about *Little House on the Prairie.*
While I loved the '70s *Brady Bunch* family, I had a certain
longing for life on the prairie, simple times with Ma, Pa, Mary,
Laura, and even sassy mean girls like Nellie. Bedtime in the
little house was one of my favorite parts. Mary and Laura
brushed their long, luxurious locks of hair and put a ruffled
sleeping cap on their heads. I wanted to be just like them. I
had worn a similar cap in my scout troop, which we had made
in celebration of the Bicentennial, and on occasion I actually
wore it to bed. *Yes, I was an unusual kid.* While I tossed the
sleeping cap aside after a few restless nights, I have for as long
as I can remember, brushed my hair at bedtime. I'm not sure if
it was because of Mary and Laura, or more because my thick
hair gets quite tangled throughout the day. It's part of my
nighttime routine — washing my face, brushing my teeth, and
finally, sitting down on my vanity stool and brushing out the
tangles as I reflect on my day. I had a busy weekend. Busy is
good for me. I saw a lot of people over the weekend, each and
every one thoughtfully asked how I am doing. When I answer
that I am doing well, sometimes people look puzzled. But,
remember…I choose happy, so even when I'm not, I try to
believe *(and convince others).* Not that I'm counting, but this
weekend, six people responded "Really?" when I said I was
doing fine. Still not wanting to dwell on sadness, I answered,
"Yes, I'm doing okay." To which they then responded, "Well,
you look good." *I suppose I do look good.* My body has been
through an awful lot in the past two months, but I don't quite
yet look like a sick person, and certainly not someone who has
cancer. My busy weekend kept my anxieties about this
coming week to a minimum. And yet tonight, as I got ready
for bed, it hit me — hard. As I brushed my hair, I realized that
maybe I am not really doing as well as I want to believe. The

tears started and haven't yet stopped. I don't want to believe it's about the hair. Just recently, in a store that specializes in items for cancer patients, a clerk blurted out "I love your hair." Usually, compliments embarrass me, but I answered back, "I love my hair, too. I won't have it in a few more weeks." The poor woman didn't know what to say. She quietly answered, "It looks so — soft." My hair is soft. My hair was once a silky blonde just like Mary's on Little House. Although some coarse gray graces my temples from raising three teenagers, the rest of my hair truly is a lovely texture. And tonight, as I brushed it, I cried. Even the anticipation of pretty scarves, hats, and silly wigs that thrill my first graders does not take away the true sadness I feel about losing my hair. Yes, it's just hair. It will grow back. But in the meantime, I won't look so good. I will look like a sick person. I will look like someone who has cancer. When people ask me how I am doing, I will still probably answer, "I'm doing well," and they will wonder, as will I...*REALLY*?

The wisdom in this story: Even in Walnut Grove, there was sickness and sadness. As Mary had to accept that she was becoming blind, I have to accept that I have cancer. (Kevin Hagen, the actor who portrayed) Doc Baker, who lovingly made house calls on Little House on the Prairie died of cancer in 2005. Cancer sucks.

The Team

Tuesday, December 8

It is said that when a person is blind or deaf, the other senses are more prominent. I have decided that when a person has cancer, all five senses explode. The world becomes brighter and louder. The antiseptic smell of hospitals becomes unforgettable. Each bite of food before treatment is delectable, as one never quite knows when medicine may affect taste buds or induce the onset of nausea. Every gentle touch warms the heart. Yes, my senses are exploding. Tonight, I attended a basketball game. I didn't feel like being there. I still have discomfort from my port. Yet, my daughters were cheering, and of course I didn't want to miss it. The gymnasium lights were bright. The sneaker skids across the floor were loud. The smell *(well, it was boys' basketball – and teenage boys smell)*. My husband and I had gone out for a nice dinner before the game, and while I enjoyed every bite of my meal, my stomach felt a little bit unsettled. As I literally leaned on my sweet husband, the closeness felt comforting. He has been unbelievable. All of this is a struggle for him, too. He is a good man. He appears almost helpless. It's sad. He wants to "*do*" and yet I'm having trouble letting go of my independence. Together, we are an amazing duo. We don't quite start and finish each other's sentences, but he is my world. We just fit. We're the typical happy family, three kids and a dog, wait three kids and three dogs. *(My son calls the two puppies our mid-life crisis dogs)*. Yes, life is good. So, back to basketball. I admit to having a favorite player. His brother played football with my son, and I have watched him grow up on the basketball court throughout the past four years. Nothing ever seems to break him. He is confident without being arrogant, talented without stealing the limelight, and focused – always focused on the game. He is an amazing player. Tonight, amidst the loud sneaker skids some boys fell to the ground, my favorite player staring up at the bright gymnasium lights. When he stood, he appeared to shake his head briefly. *(I wondered if he was trying to shake off the injury, or if perhaps he had the wind knocked out of him a bit).* Then there was blood. It appeared that an opponent's head had hit his chin, and he was whisked off to the athletic trainer's office. He wasn't gone long, but as the scoreboard reflected, the minutes of the game kept ticking along. Perhaps it was my imagination, but the team didn't seem to have their same momentum without him. He returned, with what appeared to be steri-strips on his chin, and was right back in the game— and he was on fire. He got knocked down another time or two, and each time got up with a more intense, focused look. To put it bluntly, he looked a little pissed. The team *(more together when he was back in the game)* was ready to win. For a brief moment, I questioned *What if they lose? What if they lose because he was off the court momentarily?* I wanted that win more than anything—just for him. It was a close game, but they did it...57-54. I want to be that player. I want to be confident, focused, and amazing. I want to shake off the pain. In life, the minutes of the day don't stop because I am sick. Life goes on, whether I'm in the game, or sidelined. My family is my team. They don't seem to have the same momentum without me. I want to be on fire. I've gotten knocked down a time or two, and I desperately try to stay intensely focused on fighting for the win. To put it bluntly, I'm a little pissed. Cancer is ugly— incisions, steri-strips, a medi-port, chemo, and radiation. Yet, my senses are exploding with all that is good and right in my life...gym shoes and all.

The wisdom in this story: We will get through this, and my family will be just fine, even if I need to rest momentarily.

Please Don't Worry

Wednesday, December 9

For all who read my stories—please don't worry about me. In spite of the sadness in my stories and the jelly donut days, I actually am doing quite well. I feel the power of the many prayers coming my way, and have trust in my doctors and faith in my treatment plan. So, why do I write, and why is it often sad? A dear retired teacher friend and breast cancer survivor painted during her treatments. She encouraged me to do something to help myself with the wide range of emotions I would experience. Since I can't even paint a paint-by-number, I chose to write. Writing has been very cathartic for me, and the words flow freely. While my initial intent was simply to update others on surgery dates and treatments, it has become my very personal narrative. Others have encouraged me to publish a book, and I am quite serious about pursuing that idea when my story has a happily-ever-after kind of ending. I want to publish, because my stories are real. One thing I have learned about the breast cancer world, is it's all about the "fluff." Everyone wants it to be pink and pretty. You will be cured. Very few people want to tell you about the emotional stuff, the medical stuff, the scary stuff, the real stuff. My biggest challenge in all of this has been the fear of the unknown. With each hurdle, I look back and I'm able to say I survived that fill in the blank *(emotional thing, medical thing, scary thing)*. My stories are something I would want to read if I were a newly diagnosed cancer patient. It's all out there. No secrets—raw emotion and the real truth. If I am able to publish my book, it just might help make someone else's journey a little easier. That alone, would bring me great joy. SO, even though sometimes I whine and cry a lot in my stories, and sound like I'm ready to jump off the deep end, I truly am okay. *(Yes, sometimes I have to say that 100 times to convince myself, but I am okay)*. In the event I ever feel that I'm

78

not, I've learned in the medical world there is always a pretty little white *happy pill*. Nope, I haven't needed the little white pill yet. As my Southern friend would say, "Y'all are my therapy." So as you read, please don't fret. Don't feel that you wish you could do something for me but are unable. While the miles may separate us, your warm thoughts never do. Family, friends, and even strangers have reached out to our family in ways I never would have expected. I have gotten to the point that I'm not afraid to ask if I need something, and gosh that feels good. We are well-cared for and loved deeply. Being there by my side, reading my stories, and leaving notes of encouragement help me tremendously. But don't ever feel sorrow when you read my stories. This whole big, long novel will have a happily-ever-after kind of ending. It just might take awhile...

The wisdom in this story: "A strong person is not the one who doesn't cry. A strong person is the one who cries and sheds tears for a moment, then gets up and fights again."
(unknown)

Ready or Not

Thursday, December 10

I don't dwell on my childhood. Really, I don't. I have a pretty awesome adult life to live and for which to be thankful. Yet, during this cancer journey, my mind often travels to childhood days. I had an incredibly wonderful childhood. We lived in a great neighborhood with great kids. The highlight of most summer nights was flashlight tag. Two boys in our neighborhood had early bedtimes and were seldom *(in my memory anyway)* allowed to play flashlight tag. My sister and I were out there—every game. There were probably about 8 of us, maybe 10. One of us stood in the neighbor's driveway, under the safe warm glow of the light, and counted. Everyone else ran to hide. It's a simple game, yet when I mentioned it to someone a few years ago, they had never heard of it. The shout of "ready or not, here I come" alerted all who were hiding that the "seeker" was coming to look for you. I often stood right at my neighbor's back door, the one that led into the garage. I wanted to be the first to be found. Sometimes I hid a bit further away, but was terrified they would forget to find me. I can still remember my heart beating faster, and the fear I felt during that game. The shout of *"all-ee, all-ee, all-ee, all come free"* was the signal that they had decided to stop looking for you and that you were to return to home base. I remember feeling so very relieved when I heard that call. I'm not sure what I was afraid of...the dark, being alone, or not being discovered quickly enough, but I was afraid. I was glad to be able to play, but sometimes wished that like the two boys who weren't allowed to play, my mom would stand at the door and call for me to come inside. I didn't really want to be out there, but I didn't want to admit that I didn't like the game. I wanted to be brave. My mother was the best mother in the world. She was brave. Years later when my mother was going for chemo, I was a young adult, a mom of two. During her illness, my father was a wonderful caregiver. He never allowed himself to have a break. So, for one of her chemo appointments, I took the day off work. I wanted to surprise her, to take her to the appointment. When I showed up at the house, and told her why I was there, she started to cry. "No, you're not taking me," she said. "It's an awful, awful place. I don't want you to ever have to go there." And if there is anything my mother was, she was ALWAYS no matter my age, the boss of me. If mom said I didn't go, I didn't go. I didn't take her that day, yet now it's my turn to be brave. I have my very own appointments at the awful, awful place. When I first went there, I wanted to be optimistic, *(those who read my stories regularly know that I have nothing good to say about hospitals, maybe an oncology office would be better).* However, I agree with my mom. It is an awful, awful place. Rows of recliner chairs and IV drips, people in various stages of frail, from newly diagnosed to dying. And the hats — everywhere you look, there are baskets of donated knitted hats, just another reminder about the hair. Yet, it is the place where I will get better. For mom, there wasn't going to be a getting better *(Stage 4 Colon Cancer)* and I think she knew that. I will get better. Ready or not, here I come. I'm not sure what I am afraid of — three hours of medication, the ability to look at others without sad eyes, or the potential side effects that may follow — but I am afraid. I really don't want to be there, but I want to be brave. Someday, when the chemo countdown is over, I will be free.

The wisdom in this story: Even the kindest, most gentle doctors and nurses who lovingly care for their patients can't make up for an awful place.

Chemo, Cream Puffs, and Lemon Bars

Thursday, December 10

Well, I did it! Chemo #1 is complete! Yes, it was an awful, awful place, but my nurse was lovely, and I didn't have to sit in the big row of recliners. My husband was along and they escorted us to a room with two recliners. My husband called it a Chemo Suite. He made me laugh. Some patients have a negative reaction to chemo drugs — immediately. I thought for sure I'd be *that patient*. But nothing. The pre-drug "cocktail" and both chemo drugs dripped their way into my body with only a sleepy side affect. I was supposed to be there three hours, but some minor issues *(a seeping, but not quite infected port incision and an IV bag that wasn't dripping properly delayed us)* and we were there for almost five hours, but all went well. I cried only a few tiny tears, and my husband used his handkerchief a bit catching up on several pages of my stories. They allowed me to choose from a selection of beautiful knit hats and then also suggested a fleece sleeping cap to keep my head warm when I lose my hair. They also very highly recommended the slippers, and told us that the lady who knits them loves when her products are taken. I came home to a lovely front porch surprise from my best friend since ninth grade. She had been to the bakery. When I opened the box, I cried the biggest tears of my day — cream puffs and lemon bars. Throughout my growing up years, my mother always made cream puffs and lemon bars. I loved to help mommy, and she told me that my lemon bars always tasted better than hers. They really didn't, but as a mom, she always did everything to make me shine. As for the cream puffs, those were always my husband's favorite, and my mother made them especially for him. She adored him. Turns out, she was an excellent judge of character! I adore him, too — and then some. Also in the box were cannoli, and the most beautiful raspberry cake piled high with fluffy icing. What a treat! So

82

far, no signs of nausea and aside from being tired, it has been a good day. Like Santa, I'm going to settle down for a long nap. My tired eyes twinkle, my dimple is merry, my cheeks are like roses *(steroids do that)*, and my nose like a cherry. I don't have a beard or a pipe, but I have a round face and a belly full of cream puffs and lemon bars *(I already indulged in one of each!)*. I continue to be deeply touched by the kindness of others. Once again, my sister's words echo in my ears..."one day at a time." And I rocked this day! Remind me of that when I'm throwing up tomorrow.

The wisdom in this story: When life gives you lemons, find a good friend, a bakery, and a lemon bar. We're all too busy these days to make them from scratch!

Kidnapped

Friday, December 11

Sometimes, when you are 14-years-old and your mother has cancer, you get kidnapped from school to go to the nail salon. After chemo yesterday, and an appointment for an injection today, I was ready for a jelly donut kind of day. The tears were seconds from flowing, but even with the anti-nausea meds, a jelly donut didn't sound appealing. My husband and son were working, my oldest daughter was on a field trip, and I needed to be with family. So I did what any educator-mom would do, I stole my youngest daughter from school. I did follow correct protocol by calling to let them know she was needed for an "appointment." I swore her to secrecy, and yet here I am writing about it publicly. She is a perfect-attendance kind of kid. She missed part of a math class and a study hall, and I got her back just a few minutes late for cheerleading practice. *Yes, um, late to cheerleading practice.* But it was a moment we needed. It's not something I do...allowing my kids to miss school or practice when they aren't sick. Yet her world has changed a little lately, and today was a day we both needed. My excuse form to the school on Monday will say "appointment," but I will probably leave out the part about "at the nail salon." I can also legally write family emergency/personal and quite frankly I think today fit right into that category. She wasn't quite sure what to think of me. Teachers' kids tend to be rule followers. They work hard in school, they are respectful, and they do their homework on time, *usually*. She knew deep in her heart what we were doing was wrong, but yet it felt so right. She was giggly. I love giggles. Today was a day we will remember forever. And if someone dares to share my story with the school, it's really okay. I have decided that in the world of cancer, a single unexcused absence really isn't a big deal.

The wisdom in this story: Sparkly pink toes are even more perfect than a jelly donut.

Chemotherapy

Saturday, December 12

When you are a kid, it's hard to wait for Christmas. When you are a newly treated cancer patient, it's hard to wait for chemotherapy side effects. You know what *could* come, you pray it doesn't, and yet it's a little hard to live your normal life in case it does happen. You already read the disclaimer that this site is about bras, boobs, and biopsies. Let's add to that bathroom stuff. My mother suffered terribly with diarrhea and vomiting while receiving chemotherapy treatments. She ended up being hospitalized due to dehydration. I expected the same. To be honest, I was terrified. It may come, but not yet. My oncologist told me not to expect the worst, that medical advancements have come a long way since my mom's passing in 2001. Several have asked how I am doing. I'm doing okay. I don't feel my best, but I suppose that is to be expected. I have a headache. I'm tired, and it's an odd sort of foggy tired. My muscles and joints ache, and my energy level is low. My stomach isn't quite right, but I'm not *sick.* My mind seems to tell me a little which food choices look okay, and which ones don't look appealing at all. That helps. I'm taking anti-nausea pills regularly. So as I wait to see just how the chemo drugs may affect me, it's been an on-the-couch kind of weekend, and I'm not an on-the-couch kind of girl. I was able to make it to the girls' District cheerleading competition, but I missed the State Semi-Final football game. I listened to it on the radio and cried when I heard the marching band play *Go, Eagles, Go!* In my mind, I could see my spirited daughters dancing to the familiar song and I cried some more. I wanted to be there, but because of cancer, I couldn't. Cancer sucks. But I have some great friends, and they filled my day by texting me beautiful pictures of my girls... enough to fill an album. I am so richly blessed. It was a rough game — our team lost 24-7. There were some thoughts that the referees didn't seem fair. Their players

86

were huge, and four of our players sustained injuries. Once again, I see an analogy in my cancer fight and these young, talented athletes. Like referees, cancer isn't always fair. Like our oversize opponents, cancer is huge, and I already have four battle scars to prove it. Yet, like those big strong young men that live for Friday Night Lights, I will fight this battle. I will get knocked down, but I will get up again, ready to win. Today, I want to be at church to see them light the third Advent candle. I want to go Christmas shopping with my sister, nieces, and daughters. Cancer thinks otherwise. I had a restless night and it will be a couch day. I need to save my energy for a full week of work. I've said it before, and I'll say it again...*this is hard.* In my stronger moments, I look back at my September 24 mammogram date and recognize how much I have already bravely endured. Exactly three months later, it will be Christmas Eve, and I'll have many reasons to celebrate.

The wisdom in this story: Sometimes, even when you are a grownup, it's hard to wait for Christmas.

Toddlerhood

Sunday, December 13

Toddlerhood. We've all been there, done that, and some of us have even raised toddlers. Toddler tantrums. It's that brief moment in time when toddlers cannot control their emotions and frustrations. They simply explode. Those toddler behaviors return in some adults with cancer. I'm one of those adults. Bless my dear husband for dealing with me. Toddler tantrums are the absolute worst. In the midst of them, you wonder if you'll ever survive, but when they're over you can even laugh a little. Tonight was one of those nights. While I'm slightly embarrassed to be writing about it, if my stories someday become a book and help someone else with cancer feel *normal* it will be worth my blushing face, and my face is still rosy from the steriods anyway. I was correct to assume that my minimal side effects from chemo this weekend were too good to be true. As I worried about mouth sores, my husband confirmed flashlight in hand that I have a large swollen tonsil and the start of an ulcer. I was upset. As he carefully delivered the baking soda, salt, and mug to the bathroom, I started to cleanse and dress my port incision for bedtime. In the bathroom that I so meticulously cleaned this morning, *cleaning is good therapy for me,* I could not locate the non-stick bandage pads. I had boxes of gauze, but not a non-stick pad in sight. They had been on the counter this morning, and I think in my foggy state, I threw them all away with some empty contact lens boxes. Trying to be helpful, my husband began looking in the closet. I knew they weren't there. I told him, "Never mind, I'll deal with it." Without even realizing my words, I took a deep breath and blurted, "I'm sorry. I'm just pissed at the bandages. I'd rather be pissed at the bandages than pissed at the cancer." Those words made no sense. A deep breath of a sob that even surprised me emerged from myself, and a gentle pat on the back from him.

And then it was over. An unpacked grocery bag with a brand new box of non-stick pads, that I had forgotten I'd purchased, was the remedy for my incision need. I am now tucked into my nice warm bed, and thankful that raising three toddlers has helped my husband to understand my current insanity. While I know that it's cleansing to cry, I end up with sore, swollen eyes afterward and feel worse. I think that's why I tend to bottle things up inside and then like a toddler, it all just comes pouring out. Tomorrow will be a better day.

The wisdom in this story: I'm pissed at the cancer.

Only at _____ _____ High School

(*I'm not sure their privacy really deserves to be respected, but in an effort to be politically correct, I have omitted the name of the school).

Monday, December 14

And the school called me to question her absence! To be honest, I find it almost laughable that a principal would actually request that a secretary call me to find out what was meant by appointment/family-personal on my daughter's excuse blank. My tax dollars at work, scrutinizing the absence of someone in a class size of 600+ who seldom misses school. Apparently my note confused them. So which was it, an appointment, or family-personal? Well, my daughter wrote appointment when she signed herself out, so in keeping consistent, I used the same wording. It was really no one's business what type of appointment, so I left it at family-personal. To be honest, I think the secretary was a bit uncomfortable when I told her about my cancer diagnosis and mentioned that our family is struggling. Our conversation was awkward. *Cancer does that.* I told her I didn't think that an excuse of family-personal was allowed to be questioned by the district. I told her to mark it unexcused if Mr. Principal had a problem. But here is what I didn't say:

Dear _____ _____High School,

Chemo or no chemo---your district is a pain in the ass. I cannot even fathom that you employ enough individuals to have taken the time to question this early dismissal. Sometimes families deserve privacy, and sometimes families have secrets. Perhaps next time my daughter misses school, I won't call or send an excuse at all. I'll tell her to walk right out the door. My son did that once. Thankfully, he graduated already and there's not a damn thing you can do about it.

Respectfully,

Mama B.

The wisdom in this story: The school is full of drugs, alcohol, and sex. And yet, the honor-roll kid who misses part of math class and a study hall to hang out with her sick mom is the one they're worried about. Go figure.

I Get Knocked Down

Thursday, December 17

Exactly one week ago, I entered the oncologist's office, terrified about my first chemotherapy infusion. All went well. No immediate reactions, a suggestion to drink a lot and rest over the weekend. *I can do this...were my thoughts.* Saturday passed without incident, and Sunday was not too bad either. I was thrilled. Most people say that the second day after infusion is the worst. That would have been my Saturday. Then again, if you read all of my other stories, I am not the patient who follows the statistics. Monday hit me like a ton of bricks. I ached everywhere. While the nausea medications kept me from vomiting, I was right on the brink. I was hot, then cold, and simply exhausted. I struggled to get through my work day, and requested a substitute for Tuesday. On Monday night, I was in bed covered with five blankets. Even my heated mattress pad didn't bring me warmth. Then it occurred to me. My throat hurt, too. I have felt this way before. Maybe, I have strep *(which commonly afflicts first grade teachers).* A normal patient would have promptly gone to a walk-in clinic and walked out with a prescription. But, now I'm a cancer patient. My oncologist's list of reasons to call the doctor included chills and shakes. I called. Even though my temperature was hanging right around 99.8, the doctor sent me to the Emergency Room. It seems that sometimes with chemo, the chills might indicate low white blood cell count regardless of temperature. There was still some question about the possibility of infection in my port, too. So, off we went. Two attempts to access the port for blood, many vials from my arm, and a throat culture took three hours. *We will call you with the results.* They prescribed an antibiotic for strep just in case and sent me on my way. While I must say, the new hospital is beautiful, I've never heard of place that doesn't have a rapid strep test. My culture would need to be sent out

92

to be tested. So, I was sent home wondering why I felt so crappy. I'm the not-so-patient-patient and I like answers. What was making me feel so horrible? Was it strep, something with which I've dealt with countless times throughout my career? Or was it the chemo? If it was strep, that meant that I'd survived the chemo just fine with minimal side effect. If chemo, well....I'm in for a long haul. I waited patiently for a phone call on Tuesday. Nothing. Results still pending. My bowels became upset *(as I still can't quite decide if I need the stool softener or the anti-diarrheal)*. Were my bowels upset because of the chemo, the anti-diarrheal, or even yet another side effect from taking an antibiotic? I cried, and decided that even a single dose of anti-diarrheal wasn't for me. I went to work on Wednesday. It was a little rough. It crossed my mind that perhaps my electrolytes were dipping overnight, and I drank almost a whole bottle of nasty purple sports drink. As the day went on, I seemed to feel better. After work, I rested a bit, and went to visit my favorite hairstylist for a sassy new short haircut. I decided that going short first would make going bald appear less drastic. She couldn't have been sweeter. I have gotten short haircuts before, so it really wasn't a huge deal. My last short haircut was when I was busy with a New York City trip with my daughters, and my son's prom and graduation. I remember I kept telling her back then, "Go shorter, I don't know when I'll have time to take care of my hair." So this time, it truly wasn't bad. I just pretended I was getting my cute short haircut for fun, and we enjoyed catching up with one another. When she and her sister told me "no charge" at the checkout, "this is what we do," I felt my eyes fill with tears. As I hugged my dear stylist and friend of 16 years, I whispered into her ear, "I hate cancer." Yes, it sounds cliche, but I bare my soul to my hairdresser. She promised a house call when I'm ready for a buzz cut, and we hugged again. I told her, "We did good—we didn't even cry." As I walked out the door into the the still-balmy December evening—I fell. Flat. On. My. Face. I didn't feel myself tripping. I don't remember going down. I do remember the feeling of pavement on my face, and feeling like I hurt everywhere. A sweet lady offered to help me up, and I kindly asked that she get my hairstylist for me. I don't remember a man helping me up, but I do remember the worried looks and flurry of ice packs that followed. A swollen hand, swollen lip, lost contact lens, sore arm, sprained ankle, and scraped leg did manage to distract me momentarily from the word cancer. *Cancer sucks, but so does falling.* My husband and son came to get me and my van. My son drove me home. It was hard. He told me it was okay to cry. This wonderful young man I've spent 20 years trying to protect, now comforting me. I fell apart, as much as a mother actually allows herself to fall apart in front of her son. He brought me in the house, cleansed my wounds, covered me with ice packs and tucked me into bed. I raised a good man. Today is a new day. I hurt everywhere. Tonight, I'll attend my girls' Holiday Concert at school, which will lighten my mood and help me feel ready for Christmas. But somewhere, in my mind, I will be humming a song I sometimes hear on the radio — "I get knocked down, but I get up again." *(Chumbawamba)*

The wisdom in this story: Some people say the second day after chemo is rough. In my opinion, the whole week is a little rough.

The Applause

Sunday, December 20

When my oldest daughter was a toddler, she fell — a lot. She desperately tried to keep up with her active big brother, but try as she might, her tiny legs just wouldn't allow it. Each time she went down, she hesitated a bit, and then tears...big tears from her even bigger, beautiful blue eyes. Then it was over. Always eager to please, she smiled, even giggled while the tears were still flowing. It once occurred to me that during that time of hesitation, she was watching for our reaction to her fall, and the emotions followed accordingly. If we flinched, sighed, or expressed concern, she cried. However, if we kept on smiling, she did, too. We knew she was going to fall, and lovingly awaited each tiny crash. Sadistic as it sounds, we applauded when she fell. The result...fewer tears. As I entered into my first chemo, I desperately wanted to keep up, but try as I might my body just wouldn't allow it. With each low-grade temp, ache, spasm, dizzy, lightheaded, nauseous moment, and the big fall, I felt defeated and big tears fell from my eyes. I wanted to be my happy self, a pleaser. Everyone told me attitude was everything. People told me I might not even have side effects. I wanted to be able to handle chemo and keep on smiling. I didn't want chemo to interfere with the way I live my life. Yet, chemo stopped me, and I was deeply disappointed. I thought I could do it, but I felt defeated, and this was only round #1. Then came the applause. When I went for my chemo follow-up appointment, my nurse (*the best-nurse-in-the-world*) asked me how I was doing. When I told her chemo had kicked me, she quietly answered, "I thought it might. The steroids wore off and you crashed. It happens." My nurse, someone in a position of medical authority, validated that it was truly okay to feel awful. She had expected me to crash. It happens. Chemo does that. It wasn't because of my efforts or attitude.

My body just simply couldn't handle it. The physician's assistant confirmed that I deserved to feel less than my normal. She also gently cautioned that it could get worse. I asked if I could just stay on steroids for the course of my treatment. Apparently that isn't a medical option. A drop in blood pressure or blood sugar may have caused my lightheadedness and fall. A change in my blood pressure medication and suggestion to add sugar and calories to my diet may help improve how I feel. This week should be better. She said the week before chemo is the best—and then they knock you down again. At least this time, I'll know a little more what to expect. Instead of trying to work, missing work, trying to work, and missing again, I will give myself an extra two days off before I return. And while I have many who are applauding me along the way, my nurse's validation that it's okay to feel awful will stay close in my heart. I don't think anyone expected me to get through chemo without a struggle. Yet, that is what I expected of myself.

The wisdom in this story: I crashed, but it really wasn't my fault.

Fashion Show

Wednesday, December 23

When I was a teenager, I was a shopper! I was a bargain shopper, and never bought a thing that wasn't on sale, but I had a beautiful wardrobe. One of the best things about those marathon-shopping-trips with my mom was to come home and try it all on again. I had a fashion show for her, proudly modeling each outfit. I wore a size one *(wow, really)* and I had a great eye for color. It was the '80s. We were born to stand out. Fast-forward 30 years. I no longer admit my real size to anyone, not even myself. I wear *mom clothes:* practical shoes, dress pants, knit shirts, and teacher cardigans...brown, black, khaki, and grey. And now pink — *lots of pink.* I live vicariously through my own teenagers who each have their own unique sense of fashion. My oldest daughter always color-coordinates everything — down to the jewelry. I sometimes joke that she dresses better for a day in high school than I do to go to work. My younger daughter can pair the craziest combination of things and pull it off. She, too always looks great. When you have two teenage daughters who also like to have fashion shows, you don't shop much for yourself. Essentials--I buy the essentials. Lately, essentials have included a wide assortment of scarves and hats. I have worn some of the pretty scarves around my neck, which reminds me of the popularity of scarves in my early teaching days. It seems scarves have returned, with many ways of tying them around one's neck. Soon, I'll learn to tie them around my head. I have never liked hats. My sister is a hat girl, she looks adorable in a hat on a bad hair day or lounging by her pool. Me, the visors bother me, and frankly I think I look silly. But, now I have hats. A cap here and there, and some light winter hats for when our winter weather will finally turn cooler. However, my most exciting recent purchase is a box of bandeaus in a wide range of colors...some really wild colors. The company describes the bandeau as the perfect accessory for girls who love to try out new styles. It advertises 11 different ways to wear the bandeau. My youngest daughter agreed to model all 11 ways for me. The first two ways resembled traditional headbands, there were three ways to wear it around your neck, three ways to wear it as a full head-covering, one as a ponytail wrap, and one that looked a little pirate-like. The final *(and funniest)* way to wear the bandeau, was as a shirt. As my tiny, size *zero* daughter wiggled her way into the bandeau, she even agreed that it looked a little ridiculous. I marveled that she could actually make it fit, as even my size one 1980's body wouldn't have fit into a bandeau. At my current size, perhaps it would make a good knee wrap, *a good thing to keep in mind if I happen to fall again.* After her fashion show, the stylish bandeaus were placed back in the box. I was determined that I wouldn't try on anything until I had a need. It will soon be time. They told me I would lose my hair three weeks after my first chemo treatment. "Not MY hair, I commented...I have really thick hair. My mother never lost all of her hair with chemo." "Yes," the doctor patiently repeated..."you will lose *all* of your hair. It has nothing to do with the kind of hair. It's the combination of drugs we will be giving you. You will lose your hair. Plan for it about three weeks after your first treatment." So I planned for three weeks, but like everything else, I don't do things like everyone else. Exactly 10 days after my first chemo, I noticed my hair was falling out. I didn't tell anyone. I was a bit in denial. Perhaps it wasn't. But yes, it was. I noticed a little more each day. This morning, only 13 days after my first chemo, my hair started coming out in large chunks. I told my husband, my co-workers, and my non-shedding dogs, *thank heavens my dogs don't shed, too.* I didn't tell my kids. I'm not ready for a fashion show yet. But on this eve before Christmas Eve, my house is quiet. I may head back to my bedroom a little early. I may slip a bandeau onto my head, just to try the different styles. I want to be prepared for three weeks after my first chemo, the day I suspect I may be totally and completely bald.

I think the bandeau will be the perfect accessory to my mom wardrobe when I go for chemo #2. After all, I was a teenager in the '80s. I was born to stand out.

The wisdom in this story: My mom in Heaven has the best view for my bandeau fashion show. She will love my new look.

A Clipper Cut for Christmas

Friday, December 25

While a few people think my son looks like his dad, most people tell him that he looks just like his mama — *not exactly what a teenage boy wants to hear*. My son has beautiful hair. When he was young, big soft bangs framed his face. Never a bowl cut, but never a buzz. Scissors only for my handsome son...until he was old enough to decide. He wanted a buzz cut. My hairstylist, who has sons of her own, adored him. As he walked back to her chair, he would tell her clippers, and I shouted scissors. We managed to compromise. She scissor cut the top to keep me happy, and buzzed the back and sides especially for him. Eventually, I decided that there were bigger battles to fight, and let her clipper cut his whole head. As a high school athlete, he noticed that many of the football players clipper-cut their own hair. He wanted a set of clippers. I said no. But as big brothers often do, he turned to his littlest sister. He told her he wanted clippers for his birthday. He knew she would be persistent, and she knew I wouldn't say no. He got the clippers. For all four years of high school, my son's beautiful hair was about a half inch long. I loved that face no matter what, but I missed the hair. After graduation, my son decided to let his hair grow a bit. He returned to my favorite stylist, who now clipper cuts the back and sides, all while keeping the top a beautiful scissor cut length. She gave me a short scissor cut last week. It felt perfect. Yet it wasn't enough. Christmas Eve, not a snowflake in sight, but my hair was falling...falling out fast — big, bothersome clumps. It was much faster and far worse than I'd ever imagined. My stylist friend told me she would come to my house to shave my head when I was ready. As much as I love her, I didn't need her. My son is an expert with clippers. Today was the day. It started as a tearful moment for me, and then we laughed a little. I told him I secretly admired the girls who were bold enough in the '80s to wear the punk hairstyles. The more he clipped, the more liberated I felt. *It really is just hair.* My blue eyes glistened a little. He told me I looked good. I told him his littlest sister would probably laugh at me. He told me he thought I looked beautiful. I've never had a hairstyle without big soft bangs that frame my face. But I have bigger battles to fight, and I let my son clipper cut my whole head. When I looked in the mirror after the final buzz of the clippers, I had to fight the tears. I'm glad he owns a set of clippers. My once beautiful hair is now about a half inch long. My son loves my face no matter what, but I know he misses the hair. Someday, I'll return to my stylist. But for now, I think people will probably tell me that I look just like my son. While it's not exactly what I'll want to hear, it will be a compliment. When I think back to his high school football days, I think my hair could fit right in with the Varsity linemen. My opponent is big. I'm going for the win.

The wisdom in this story: With every surgery, procedure, treatment, and haircut, I'm one step closer to being cancer-free.

The Time of Your Life

Wednesday, December 30

Y2K — Year 2000 — Two Thousand Zero Zero. For some, the idea of Y2K caused sheer panic, for some cautious curiosity, and yet others, a reason to party. I fit into all three categories. Y2K panic *(yes, I withdrew a fairly large sum of money from the bank, because "they" said none of the ATMs or banks would be working);* Year 2000 curiosity *(yes, I truly wondered if life would change on the morning of January 1);* and Two Thousand Zero Zero a reason to party *(of course, I had a reason to party).* Backtrack to my life as a teenager in the '80s...it was one of the best times of my life. Big hair, blue eye shadow, and the preppiest clothing wardrobe you'd ever seen *(with an occasional Flashdance look thrown in for good measure).* I read books like *The Preppy Handbook* (1980), listened to Prince's *Party Like it's 1999* song (1982); watched *Flashdance* (1983), and dated a cute boy (1986) who drove an IROC-Z Camaro and then a *Little Red Corvette* (just like in that Prince song). I married him and we sold the Corvette...for something practical. *Why did we ever let life become practical?* I love music for the rhythm, and while I can sing the words to every single Rod Stewart song, I really never quite understood the lyrics to Prince's *1999* song. I loved the song, and sang loudly the only part I knew..."*Tonight I'm going to party like it's 1999*" and at some point a little later there was "*Two Thousand Zero Zero, la, la, la.*" So in 1999, I did what any young mother of two would do. I planned a party. My son was 3½ , my daughter was 15-months-old, and most nights they went to bed at 8:00 p.m.; which meant that I went to bed at 8:30 p.m. Most of my friends went to bed at 8:30. So I planned a party for parents of babies and toddlers. Invitations were sent, with specific information that kids were welcome at this party, and we were going to "Ring in the New Year" promptly at 9:00 p.m. My mother *(the party planner of all parties)* LOVED this idea, and bragged to all of her friends about her wonderfully creative daughter. While I don't remember a lot about the evening, *I HAD stayed up a bit past my bedtime*, I do recall that I wanted everything to be perfect. My girly girl daughter wore the most adorable blue plaid skirt with a glisten of silver stripe and a turtleneck and shoes to match. I no longer dressed quite so nicely, but my daughter—SHE had style---*she still does*. We had party horns and lots of eager toddlers who blew them most of the night—and I had music…of course I needed music. Auld Lang Syne was at the top of my needs for party songs, and I found it on a mixed party tape for New Year's Eve. What I didn't know was that was a new artist had only recently (1997) released a song that remains one of my favorites to this day—and I know all of the words. Green Day, had contributed to the mixed party tape their song *Time of Your Life*. I'm not sure why, but the song made me cry that night. I still cry every time I hear it. My mother had been diagnosed with Stage 4 colon cancer in May 1999 and I was understanding the fragility of life. While I wasn't fearful of the Y2K disasters predicted in the news, that very night I simply wanted to stop time. I wanted my life to remain exactly as it was at that moment *(of course with the wishes for a third child in the future)*. As I reflect back on the past 15 years, I have to say that life has been good to me. Even with my mother's passing and my breast cancer diagnosis, life is still good. I am blessed with good friends and an incredible family. My experience with cancer has been a bit like Y2K. At first, it caused sheer panic *(This is MY awful. Why me? Why even cancer?)*; Then I became cautiously curious *(How much will I have to endure? Can I do it? What will come next? Will the cancer come back?)* And yet still, I have reason to party. Chemo round #2 for me is tomorrow—New Year's Eve *(in the morning)*. I told my nurse we would party together *(even though the chemo infusion makes me sleepy, foggy, and sort of sad)*. I'm going to party like it's 1999. My sweet daughter helped me to craft gift boxes for the patients, nurses, and doctors, gifting each with hand sanitizer and a chocolate truffle. I'm not sure about all chemo patients, but I can still eat chocolate. I have some New York City shower gel, lotion, and a party hat for my nurse. *Oh, how I would love to be in New York City!* But, I will go to the oncology office, spend several hours with my nurse *(and my sweet husband)*, and come home to my recliner chair. I hope to cook some of our New Year's Eve favorites, even though I won't be able to enjoy them. And just like in 1999, I will be ringing in the New Year at 9:00 p.m., fast asleep in my recliner. I'm sure my family will wake me at midnight, and I'll hug and kiss to *Auld Lang Syne.* But as my head hits my new satin pillowcase *(great for bald people!)*, I will be singing another familiar tune:

Time of Your Life
Green Day

"Another turning point, a fork stuck in the road
Time grabs you by the wrist, directs you where to go
So make the best of this test and don't ask why
It's not a question but a lesson learned in time
It's something unpredictable but in the end is right
I hope you had the time of your life
So take the photographs and still frames in your mind
Hang it on a shelf in good health and good time
Tattoos of memories and dead skin on trial
For what it's worth, it was worth all the while

Chorus:
It's something unpredictable but in the end is right
I hope you had the time of your life."

Ironically, the original title of this song was *Good Riddance.* Oh, how I will someday enthusiastically say good riddance to cancer. I was stuck at a fork in the road of decision-making regarding my cancer course of treatment. Time grabbed me by the wrist *(as did my surgeon)* and directed me where to go.

Even though I still ask why, I am making the best of this test. My mind is filled with photographs and still frames of each and every moment, ready to hang on a shelf in good health and good time. Following chemotherapy, I'll earn my radiation tattoos and dead skin. But as the song says, "for what it's worth, it *will* be worth all the while. It's something unpredictable but in the end is right." *(And you know I'll have the time of my life...)*

The wisdom in this story: I hope YOU always have the time of your life.

A Day in the Life of a Chemo Patient

Saturday, January 2

There are two words *(among other obvious curse words)* that I've never allowed to be used in my home...HATE and SUCKS. Hate is a word I was never allowed to use as a child. Nothing in life could be deemed so awful that you could use the word hate, especially if it was directed at another person. *Although I do recall my mother during her cancer years occasionally uttering the word hate.* I'm not quite sure when the word *sucks* became common in society, but I never liked the sound of it either. I once gently admonished a young sixth-grade boy *(not my son)* for using that word in my home. He apologized profusely for not respecting our house rules, and promised he would never ever say it again. After he left, I apologized to my own son for my teacher voice having kicked in during his friend's visit. My son *(even mature at the tender age of 11),* told me he was glad I corrected the kid. By eighth grade, the boys parted ways and that dear young man I once loved like a son chose a rather troubled path of drugs and alcohol. While no parent is ever to blame for the horrible things in our society, I wondered a little if he may have chosen a different path had someone in his own home consistently chosen to correct his inappropriate behaviors. My behaviors have been less than appropriate lately, and the words hate and sucks *(among other obvious curse words)* fill my head. While I'm well-mannered enough to not allow them to slip into my vocabulary *(except during the occasional private temper tantrum),* the words are there. In the beginning, I called those days *"Jelly Donut Days,"* but chemo changes the taste of everything, and even a jelly donut doesn't help. And so, I write. It seems safe. For those who care to follow my stories, they know I'm a good person with a big heart. They know words like hate and sucks are not all-consuming in my life. *And yet, cancer is all-consuming.* Even on my good days, it's sometimes all I think about. A friend recently said, "I can't imagine what you are going through." It was a lovely, kind comment that left me speechless. I didn't know what to say to her. Sometimes even I can't imagine what I am going through. At first, the medical part seemed the worst. While I still *hate* everything medical, the emotional stuff just really *sucks*. I'm not depressed, but there are times when there's a sadness that's just really tough to shake. While I would never want another soul to have to walk in my shoes, a simple glimpse into a day of a chemo patient may make one more tolerant of our emotions. With my first chemo treatment, they told me two days after chemo would be the worst. Last time it wasn't. My bad day wasn't until day 5. Today is now two days after round #2. It feels like the worst.

2AM: My head is sweating, my body is freezing. I'm nauseous and I can't sleep. Chemo *sucks*. Cancer go away. This is hard.

7AM: I don't want to get out of bed, but I know a shower will make me feel better. The shower will exhaust me, and I'll retreat to the recliner. I *hate* this.

8AM: While I know nutrition is important, eating and drinking are especially difficult. Fluids are crucial to help flush the toxins from my system and prevent dehydration. For breakfast, I settle for about five frosted mini-wheats and yet another large glass of grape juice, one of the few beverages I can tolerate. Hopefully these efforts will help my bladder and bowels work regularly as I heal.

9AM: A social media pop-up reminds me that a year ago today I took my girls on an adventure to see the LOVE statue in Philadelphia. I have no energy for those spontaneous moments now, which makes me frustrated and really sad. But today, my family is showing me the love.

10AM: We always take our Christmas tree down the day after New Year's, but today is a little more bittersweet than usual. My husband has the last remnants of Christmas swept away as I sit in my chair. The holidays were a bit surreal for me this year, and while I tried to enjoy myself, I sadly admit that I was just going through the motions.

11AM: Along with the take down of the Christmas tree comes the reality that vacation is almost over. My oldest daughter is doing homework, my youngest procrastinating. I just sent an e-mail to the parents of my students stating that my return will be delayed by two extra days, just in case. While I know this is best, it will be hard not to greet my students on the first day back.

12NOON: Within the last few weeks, my nurse and two thoughtful friends all told me about a free housecleaning service offered to chemo patients. I was proud to tell them that my husband and kids are amazing. They do a great job. My house looks better than when I am well. So while I sit here feeling somewhat lethargic, the whir of the vacuum and the light smell of dusting spray make me smile. While the cleaning service might be great for some, I am blessed to have family...*a really great family*, who takes care of things when I can't. Thank heavens I taught them the importance of keeping a tidy house.

1PM: The nausea continues, the muscle and joint aches have returned, and I am resting. In my mind, I'm out doing something fun to enjoy the sunny day; but in my reality, I drift between a foggy, sleepy state to a deep, snoring sleep. A tired old dog and two white fluffy puppies all share the couch with me. They seldom leave my side. I've gone from calling myself the crazy lady with three dogs to someone who truly believes animals know us best. My fluffy family brings me comfort on these days.

2PM: The two o'clock ring of my doorbell indicated that a delivery had arrived with a much-awaited package of photographs for my oldest daughter's scrapbook. She is a busy girl, and scrapbooking is something special we find time to do together. Although I wasn't feeling well, getting up off of the couch helped me feel normal, and normal is what I crave. So, for the next three hours, I did what I do best. I spent time being a mom. One of the hardest parts of my cancer diagnosis, is that it came this year...my daughter's senior year of high school. I never missed a thing my son's senior year, and yet because of cancer, I am missing doing things for and with my sweet girl. It's heartbreaking. I hate it. But these past few hours were wonderful, and as she heads out to the craft store for more supplies, I consider what might be tolerable for dinner as my nausea is significantly worse this time than with chemo round #1.

5PM: A few saltine crackers and some cherry 7-up seemed to help settle things, but only slightly. Soon my home will be filled with our favorite takeout pizza, which I know my sensitive body can't handle. It's a great option though for hungry teenagers, and an air freshener spray clears the scent of most food smells that linger. I never thought I'd say not having pizza *sucks*...but not having pizza *sucks*.

6PM: More scrapbooking with my favorite princess. We're on a roll! Chemo makes my vision slightly blurry the first few days, and my eyes are tearing a bit. I'm not sure if it's from the chemo, or real tears from the whirlwind of emotion I'm experiencing today.

9PM: Ready to fall into bed, and praying that tonight's sleep is a little more peace-filled than last night. One day closer to a cure...

This story has been filled with a whole lot of *hate* and *sucks* but

109

it has also been filled with a lot of love. Some of the words that I love best, from some very wise friends, follow:

"You are never alone..." *(from a former student who is now a twenty-something elementary teacher)*

"I continue to pray for peace and healing..." *(from someone who keeps me wrapped in prayer)*

"Stay properly focused..." *(from a dear friend and cancer survivor)*

"I can't imagine what you are going through..." *(from a sweet, thoughtful, sensitive friend)*

"Good morning, Sunshine..." *(from a friend who has her own struggles, yet greets me with this message almost daily)*

...and the very best words of all from my own sister: "one day at a time."

This is my journey. This is my story. Somewhere in it there is a lesson to be learned. Not all days are awful, but as I mentioned previously, cancer is often all-consuming. Even though I know that I am never alone, and many pray for my peace and healing, it is sometimes hard to stay properly focused. While few have the courage to admit it, many can't imagine what I am going through. But when someone greets you with "Good Morning, Sunshine," it's hard not to take things any way but one day at a time.

The wisdom in this story: I hate cancer. Chemo sucks. There will be times when there is a sadness that's just really tough to shake...yet I am so very blessed.

110

To My Son's Girlfriend

Sunday, January 3

It only occurred to me moments ago how silly I must have looked when you entered my home earlier today. With the bright yellow dish rag placed right on top of my bald head, I'm sure I was quite a sight. The coolness of the cloth brings comfort during chemo sweats, and helps to lighten the odor of the chemicals seeping through my pores that only I seem to notice. My appearance never deterred you from coming right over and seating yourself on the armrest of my couch. I know that for many reasons, it is hard for you to see me this way, and I just wanted to thank you for the time you spent with me. We chatted like schoolgirls about all of the kids-home-from-college gossip. It was great to talk with you. To be honest, I was never thrilled with the idea of my son having a girlfriend when you slipped into our lives two years ago. Most protective mothers don't want to share the affections of their son, or even worse yet, see their son someday brokenhearted. As yours was young love, I tried to keep my distance a bit, because I do get so terribly attached to those who enter my childrens' lives. So in case you don't know it sweet girl, I adore you. Today, your bright smile was just the medicine I needed, well, that and maybe a whole lot more anti-nausea meds. Thank you for just being you, and loving me, bright yellow dish rag and all. Although you are young, you are wise beyond your years. I love you, and I know my son does, too.

The wisdom in this story: Love knows no boundaries.
(unknown)

The Magic Wand

Wednesday, January 6

As a kid of the '70s, I didn't have electronics, but I could be busy for hours with Wooly Willy. If you grew up in the '70s and ever traveled more than an hour to get to Grandma's house, I know you had one. It was the perfect drawing toy.

According to Wikipedia:
Wooly Willy is a face printed on cardboard under a bubble of plastic filled with metal filings that could be moved with a magnetic wand to create features like beards, mustaches, and shaggy eyebrows on the cartoon face.

The product advertises Willy's Magic Personality and the feature I liked best *(I was a little OCD even then)*, was the perfectly enclosed magic wand. Even in my messy world, it never got lost. Almost two weeks ago, my son gave me a buzz cut. It wasn't bad. I looked like a bad-ass old lady. My scalp hurt. We went shorter. Finally, a third cut left only sparse patches of stubble. I avoided looking at myself and when I did catch a glimpse in the bathroom mirror, found myself apologizing to my family for my baldness. My scalp, as apparently is common with chemo patients, still hurt. Yesterday, with the most gentle of care, my dear husband took the razor to my head. I wanted it gone. Every single stubble. It felt fantastic, but I avoided the mirror. I went back to work today. The kids were happy it's finally "Hat Day Every Day" in my classroom. They were curious what was under my knit hat. They are six. I showed them my bald head and told them it was okay to giggle. We all giggled. It was a hard day working, but it was a good day. I mostly stayed in my classroom, but sweet, thoughtful co-workers made time to stop in to say hello. They told me I looked cute and complimented me on my color *(thanks mom for teaching me about great lipstick).* As I prepared for bed this evening, I looked in the mirror. For the first time in two weeks, I laughed out loud at myself. My eyes looked huge. My nose was red. My head *so* bald. I had a simple expression on my tired face. I looked like Wooly Willy. It's cold outside — the season of indoor recess. Occasionally I surprise the class with a new toy. An online retailer delivers to my school. A package will arrive for us next week — five Wooly Willy drawing toys. I suspect Willy will be popular. I won't say a word, but I'll wonder if the students will think he looks just like me.

The wisdom in this story: Maybe, even through the struggles of chemo, the magic of my personality is still there. If only I could find the magic wand...

Glass Half Full

Saturday, January 9

There is a saying about people who look at things with a glass half full (or glass half empty) attitude. The problem with sayings like that are sometimes people like me can't remember which one means optimistic. *Full is the way we want to be, right? Or is it empty?* Seriously, anytime I try to use that phrase, I can't remember—maybe because you can't have one without the other. A cancer survivor once told me I needed a goal. *My goal was to not let chemo kick me in the ass.* Perhaps my goal was a little too lofty. However, here I am 10 days out from chemo round #2, saying *"I can do this..."* The worst of round two has finally passed, and while some side effects remain to remind me that chemo drugs are still coursing through my body, I can function. It's not my normal, and some chemo patients gently tell me that it can be many months after the last chemo until my real normal returns. But it's the optimism I love that has returned. I'm back. *Kinda.* So whether it's half full or half empty, my body is there. Half of the chemo drugs I need have been infused into my body via the port I love to hate, and they are prayerfully working as they are intended. Two rounds down, two to go. Me, I'm still trying to figure out if I'm empty or full, but as I said long ago, I choose happy. I have a new goal. It is my goal to accept the fact that the next two rounds of chemo will most likely kick me in the ass, but to know that there is always some kind of wonderful waiting on the other side.

The wisdom in this story: Sometimes you really can't have one without the other.

I'm Not Going to Cry

Thursday, January 14

My son was a tough five-year-old. I remember the day he visited the pediatrician for his kindergarten immunizations. He never cried. Fast-forward two years, when it was my oldest daughter's turn. She has a September birthday, so she was young, still only four. She made the school cutoff date for enrollment, and as much as I couldn't fathom sending such a young one to school, it was a wise educational decision to send her. She was ready. According to two kindergarten teacher friends, she was more than ready. My kid, at age four, was ready to soar. But there were the immunizations. Big brother boasted and told her that he didn't cry...not one bit. She was sassy, and answered right back, I'm NOT going to cry either. As I watched her tiny body climb onto the pediatrician's table, I questioned her readiness. As the needle poked through her tender flesh, one very large tear formed in the corner of her eye. She fought hard not to blink — she would not be outdone by big brother. That big tear rolled down her cheek. One, big, lonely tear. And yes, I later allowed her to say she didn't cry. That brave young lady is now a senior in high school and has far surpassed any expectation I ever had for her, both academically and socially. She just received the Soaring Eagles award at her school.

According to the school district website,
"A student can be nominated for reasons including, but not limited to, positive attitude, noteworthy service, marked improvement, great attendance, impressive effort, academic achievement and constant excellence. Nominations are reviewed by a grade-level selection team of administrators, guidance counselors and teachers. Two students per grade level are chosen each month."

My daughter has a tender heart, and speaks openly about my

illness. She recently wanted to be sure I heard Rachel Platten's new song *Stand by You*. The stations play it often, and I think of her when I hear it.

"Hands, put your empty hands in mine
And scars, show me all the scars you hide
And hey, if your wings are broken
Please take mine so yours can open too
Cause I'm gonna stand by you
Oh, tears make kaleidoscopes in your eyes
And hurt, I know you're hurting, but so am I
And love, if your wings are broken
Borrow mine 'til yours can open too
Cause I'm gonna stand by you"
(Rachel Platten)

Today is day 15. In one week I will go for chemo round #3. The first time, I didn't know what to expect. I thought the second time would be better *(it wasn't)*. This time, I actually dread going. My wings are feeling a little broken. As I climb into the chemotherapy chair, I will question my readiness. As the needle pokes through my tender port, a very large tear will form in the corner of my eye. I will fight hard not to blink. I will not be outdone by cancer. That big tear will roll down my cheek. *One, big, lonely tear.* Then, as much as I don't want it to happen, more tears will follow. As the tears make kaleidoscopes in my eyes, I will be okay. I will know that my daughter's wings will help me to keep soaring. She's gonna stand by me.

The wisdom in this story: Tears make kaleidoscopes in your eyes. (Rachel Platton)

116

Wishes

Wednesday, January 20

When I was a kid, there was no better day in the year than my birthday. My mother had a way of making birthdays seem magical. As she tucked you into bed the night before a birthday she gently said, "you're never going to be *(insert age)* again." She loved to tell the story that at age ten, I cried at those words. I suppose I loved being ten. While the years blur together, I can recall most early birthday celebrations and cakes vividly: the circus train cake, the Snow White cake, the Holly Hobbie ice cream cakes *(there were two!)*; as well as gifts received from friends: the mouse book from Janilyn, the butterfly stick pin from Sarah, and the Pet Rock from Pam. While there may be a few photos from those occasions, we didn't document life in the '70s by snapping photographs of everything. Yet those images are crisply imprinted in my memory. Good times. Good days. Birthdays. I have another memory of a birthday that is quite bittersweet. I was 23. My grandmother had passed away shortly before and I had just returned home from her funeral. My parents stayed out of town a little longer, and my birthday was going to be uneventful. On the day of my birthday the doorbell rang, and there stood my mother's best friend, a beautiful homemade cake in hand. She spoke barely above a whisper, fighting back tears, *"Your mother wanted you to have a cake."* I don't recall the details of the moments or years that followed, because the reality of being a college grad and grownup hit me hard that year. There were 10 more years of favorite dinners *(lasagna, always mom's best lasagna)* and birthday cakes *(usually ice cream cakes)* before my mom passed away. I was 33. After my mom's death, birthdays never seemed the same. She was gone, and so was the magic. While others lovingly made attempts to make my day special, I've never fully enjoyed a birthday since. While I take a deep breath to blow out the many candles each

117

year, I can't recall the last time I made a wish. The little girl in me grew up. This year, I have a wish. Some might think I will wish for no cancer, but I'm mature enough to realize *that* requires more than a simple birthday wish. While my wish is a big one, there is a possibility that it just may come true. My birthday is just a few short weeks away and my girls will be at National Cheer Championships in Disney. I want to be there. This is their biggest moment in cheer, and my older daughter's last moment as a high school cheerleader, as she is a senior. I need round #3 of chemo to be a little more gentle on my already exhausted body. I need the side effects to be minimal and subside quickly. I need to feel well enough to travel, and book a last minute flight. If I get my wish, I will be wearing Mickey Mouse ears on my birthday, the personalized ones like I had as a kid. I will wear the big pin that proudly announces "Today is my birthday!" and I will feel ten again. My birthday will seem magical, and I will cry. I will never be 47 again. I will have a cake, and when I blow out the candles, I will make a wish. But, you see—I need to make my wish before my birthday for it to come true on time. So, I won't be wishing on a birthday candle, I'll be wishing on a star. When they access my port for chemo tomorrow, they will tell me to take a deep breath, *(they think it distracts you from the discomfort but it really doesn't)*. With that deep breath, I'll be wishing for Disney. I'll look briefly toward the heavens and know that my mother is beyond those wishing stars. And with all my heart, I will wish. Somewhere inside of me is a kid who still believes that dreams really do come true.

The wisdom in this story:
"When you wish upon a star, makes no difference who you are
Anything your heart desires, will come to you.
If your heart is in your dream, no request is too extreme
When you wish upon a star, like dreamers do."

(Leigh Harline and Ned Washington)

Pandora

Thursday, January 21

While I remember every last detail about elementary school, my middle school years were a blur. I don't think I hated middle school at the time, but now that I look back, I think I hated middle school. I lost my locker key often, I was tiny and a single-file-in-the-hallway kind of girl. The big kids and hallway chaos terrified me. I had two teachers at the middle school who were a husband-wife duo. The wife was from the Ukraine. *I wanted to send her back to the Ukraine.* Yes, she was *that* mean. But there was one, very, very special English teacher. She was a long-term-substitute and I loved her. Her name was Mrs. B and she lived in my neighborhood. I think because she knew my mom she gave me a little special attention. As a tiny, shy, quiet one who *probably hated middle school*, I am certain I needed that attention. Mrs. B taught me to diagram sentences. I did them perfectly. Everyone *hated* diagramming sentences. I *loved* diagramming sentences — *because I loved Mrs. B.* She is why I love English still today. It remained my favorite subject throughout high school, and I was a published author of a very small article in an international publication in college. At work, my coworkers affectionately used to call me *"The Queen of Bullshit"* when we were required as a team to write something pleasing to administrators. *(I've since passed that title on to a younger, more capable teacher).* My students tend to have nice scores at team data meetings, and I am convinced that it is because above all else that I do in the classroom, teaching students to write is a priority. They have voice! Anyway, Mrs. B impacted my life tremendously. When I write my cancer stories, I sometimes hesitate to use fragmented sentences, or start sentences with and, because, and but; I overuse yet and however, have run-on sentences, and use way too many commas, italics, dots, and dashes; but I believe that is what gives my stories *"voice."* It's the real stuff—no fluff, as I say! I don't know how long Mrs. B was at our school, but even then I knew how to recognize a special teacher. When she left, I organized a collection of money from the students, and my mother took a friend and I *(nope, that should be me and a friend)* to the mall. We bought a porcelain teacher figurine for Mrs. B. I was so sad to see her go. I don't remember the teacher who returned, but I remember I didn't like her. I didn't like a lot of English teachers after that...*but I loved English.* Sometime during middle school I learned Greek Mythology. I *loved* Greek Mythology. I remember Pandora's box and I remember it being evil, but that's all I remember. Present day, I hear people talk about Pandora radio and my daughters have Pandora jewelry. The names of both have always puzzled me, but never quite enough to revisit Greek Mythology. I had always admired the Pandora bracelets, but they were too cost prohibitive for my mommy budget. I splurge often for my kids, but seldom for myself. When I noticed that the jewelry store just happened to be right down the street from my oncologist, and it was Christmastime, I decided to splurge... for ME! I used money from my mother-in-law and I think she was pleased with my choice. I bought the bracelet, and my first tiny charm---a sparkly silver #1. It was my "prize" for enduring round one of chemo. My husband took me directly to the jewelry store after round two. Two was out of stock, just my luck, and I questioned *who actually buys a two?* Today I will "earn" number three, and instant gratification is nice, so I'm hoping it's in stock. I will be absolutely delighted to finally purchase number four, signifying the end of chemo. Someone asked if I will buy one for each week of radiation. I will have *seven* weeks of radiation. *A charm for each week is definitely NOT in my mommy budget.* But, my focus now is on tomorrow's number three. I can never sleep the night before chemo— yep—anxiety! So, I turn on the computer. It's a terrible idea to read online about cancer. The only truth one might find in reading about cancer is that *every patient is different. Every treatment from one to the next (even in the same patient) is different. Everything is fairly unpredictable.* There seems to be a general consensus and one also shared by my doctor, that chemo has a cumulative effect and is a little worse each time, *not something one really wants to read about either.* So I searched *Pandora.* In the myth, beautiful Pandora opened the mysterious box. Out came all the troubles known to mortals, the evils of the world, including but not limited to:

(And yes, my list is in alphabetical order – English lovers tend to like it that way!)

death
disappointment
disease
envy
hate
misery
poverty
sadness
sickness
worry

"These evils all came out, like tiny, buzzing moths. Pandora slammed the lid shut. Pandora could still hear a voice from the box, pleading to be let out. Epimetheus agreed that nothing inside the box could be worse than the horrors that had already been released, so they opened the lid once more." (Greek Mythology)

What follows, is the last part of the story that I had forgotten from my middle school days. It's the best part of the story, yet somehow the part I had forgotten: "All that remained in the box was HOPE. It fluttered from the box like a beautiful dragonfly, touching the wounds created by the evil creatures, and healing them. Even though Pandora had released pain and suffering upon the world, she had also allowed HOPE to follow them." *(From: myths.e.2bm.org because yes, my teacher also taught us not to plagiarize!)* So, that's it—HOPE! Hope will be my final Pandora charm after the many months to come, and maybe I'll even splurge for a Pandora dragonfly charm! In the meantime, I'm hoping that my childhood neighbor moms who read these stories may know the whereabouts of my beloved Mrs. B. I thought she seemed "old" when I knew her, and that was 35 years ago. But it saddens me to think about searching for an obituary. I hope I'm not too late to tell her thank you. I think she might like knowing that I am a teacher, *(and an author).*

The wisdom in this story: Even with disappointment, disease, sadness, sickness, and worry, there is always HOPE.

PS: I still couldn't sleep. I turned the computer on again. An online people search tells me Mrs. B is still gracing this Earth with her presence. If the online information is correct, she is 88 and still living in the neighborhood. She lives one block over, almost parallel to my childhood home. My house number was 5243, her house number is 5243, different streets, but cool commonality. I vaguely remember knowing that fact as a kid. As soon as my chemo side effects subside, I think I'm going to visit her. Although it's doubtful she will remember me, I can tell her that I love her.

Tough Guys Wear Pink

Saturday, January 23

As I sit inside and look out at the beautiful snow, my mind travels to a more simple day last summer. We don't vacation every year, but when we do, I cherish the calm I feel when somewhere warm and sunny. The hectic pace of life seems to stop momentarily, and the glow of sunshine on the faces of my children brings me years worth of memories. Ever since I became a mom, there have been the obligatory beach pictures, posed and perfect. They never seem perfect when we are taking them (*a boy who can't contain his silly, a middle child eager to please whose patient smile becomes tired, and a stubborn little one who refuses to smile.*) But afterward, these glimpses deep into their personalities become treasures. My favorite beach picture was taken when they were ages 2, 4, and 6. They were holding hands, down by the ocean. Big brother proudly holding the hands of his sisters, the reluctant middle child fearful of the water, and the littlest one walking somewhat wobbly in the sand. While it was admittedly a posed photo, it looked so very natural. For some reason I felt compelled to recreate that photo again this past summer. While out shopping for photo-ready clothing, I was drawn toward pink, *and this was prior to my diagnosis.* While I hesitated with the pink plaid shirt for my son, I remembered him as a shy but confident fifth grader who proudly asked me to purchase a shirt for him with the logo "*Tough Guys Wear Pink.*" I bought the pink...then and now. Our summer 2015 photograph, while admittedly posed, looked so very natural. No one knew whether to look at me, the ocean, or the seagulls on the beach, so it took awhile to get the perfect shot. There were too-tight hand squeezes, threats to throw someone in the ocean, and silly seaweed mustaches. They never stopped giggling, and I stood soaking it all in realizing I love teenagers as much as toddlers. By Christmastime, the summer memory became the perfect Christmas card, and included my new favorite quote, *"Let your faith be bigger than your fear." (unknown).* When I was first diagnosed, people told me cancer would make me stronger, make my family stronger, closer. They told me I would notice things more, appreciate things more. *Those comments seemed patronizing and even insulting to me.* There was nothing wrong with my family... just the way it was at that moment on the beach last summer. And yet months later, *cancer has made me stronger, my family stronger, closer. I notice things more, appreciate things more.* **I am stronger.** When I look back at each surgery, recovery, procedure, port access, chemo infusion, and awful side effect, I wonder how I have done so well and still found time to be mostly mom. While the months ahead frighten me, I feel I have the strength to fight this fight. My family is stronger, because as much as they rely on me, they are perfectly capable of embracing their independence when I am flopped on the couch recovering. While my family has always been close, I notice their shared conversations and giggles more often. Just like when they were toddlers, I wish I could bottle the sound of their giggles to get me through the hard days. I appreciate my wonderful husband and incredible children for surviving this journey with me. *It is hard for all of us.* I appreciate my now grown son who follows his father's lead and helps take care of me. Like that day many years ago on the beach, he reaches out to his little sisters at a time when they need him most — perhaps now more than ever. I secretly smile when I pretend not to notice the pink breast cancer awareness wristband my son proudly wears on his arm. Although I didn't need a cancer diagnosis to realize it, I couldn't have raised a better young man. Seaweed mustaches, youthful silliness and all, it really is true — tough guys wear pink. Cancer has made me stronger — my family stronger, closer. I notice things more, appreciate things more. But, still no fluff — *cancer sucks.* Two days out from chemo and I feel lousy. Sensitivity to smell, nausea, chemo body odor, muscle aches, metallic tastes, and indigestion are with me and I wait.

Tummy troubles subside with medication but only slightly and I have no appetite. It is a challenge to stay hydrated. I pray to keep only on the edge of vomiting, and am thankful for anti-diarrheal medicine *(yes, a disclaimer in a previous story reminds you there may be times I share too much information)*. I am tired, weak, and grumpy. *This is hard — much, much harder than I ever anticipated.* While I always recognize there are people whose situations are far worse than mine, *this is MY awful.* But with a loving family, a one-day-at-time attitude, and a beautiful snowfall to watch while I rest, I know that I can do this...

The wisdom in this story; I am one day closer to being cured and another summer evening on the beach.

(Note: I was able to return to the beach on July 25, six months after this story was written. My July 25 beach story ends this book.)

Blizzard Brain

Sunday, January 24

While every chemo patient experiences different side effects, the foggy effect of the first few days bothers me almost the most *(well, maybe not as much as the chemo odor)*. While I had expected nausea, vomiting, even diarrhea, I didn't know that the foggy, slightly dizzy, not quite right feeling existed. Sleep becomes deeply interrupted, and while short naps feel like long slumbers, there are other times I lie awake for hours my mind racing. My vision, while bothersome, is not quite blurry, and my eyes tear a lot. It is difficult to process thoughts, and words don't seem to come out right, except on paper which I suppose helps explain why I write. I can't even begin to describe the feeling—you're just *not there*. Life goes on around you and you're almost but not quite content to simply observe. It frustrates me terribly. While by normal standards, I was the household-managing, multi-tasking mother who worked a full-time job and still managed to love life as busy as it kept me; as a cancer patient I am a puddle of mush. I feel myself going through the motions, trying to *"be there"* but not really *"being."* Some days are a big blur of puppy snuggling, too much television, and requesting that each family member, whomever happens to pass by first bring me medicine, a drink, and yet another Italian ice. And then, it passes. I start to feel slightly normal again. While I haven't felt capable of doing one ounce of housework during chemo, *(bless my family for carrying on this task)*, it feels gratifying to pour bleach into the washing machine and wash a load of towels and washcloths, even if I do rely on a family member to put the items in and out of the washer and dryer. *I poured bleach. Yippee!* Chemo brain as I call it, passes after a few days, yet this weekend I am plagued by something worse—*Blizzard Brain*. In the midst of my chemo recovery, Mother Nature dumped down a record breaking 30+ inches of snow in our county, most within a 24-hour period. And here I sit. Snowed in. I have no desire or energy to go anywhere even if I could, but my mind is racing. I have too much time to think. Last night was more than a little rough. While being over halfway thru chemo should have me feeling confident, I am still fearful. When I questioned the doctor's report of my aggressive tumor at the start of my chemo, she carefully said four words: *bone, brain, liver, lung* – four terrifying words in a list of places that a single breast cancer cell might likely choose to go. She calmly followed those words with, "the chemo will take care of it." I felt reassured, but today, my mind is racing. I want to be *sure*. My mind is filling with *what-ifs* faster than the snowplow drivers can fill their plows. What if a cell escaped and grew into a tumor too large for this course of chemo? What if a cell hasn't yet appeared but someday will? And the hardest question of all, what if the cancer comes back again, *even years from now?* Will I finish this battle strong enough to fight again? Tears fall quickly from my eyes, but thankfully no more snowflakes fall outside. It is cleanup time. Time to dig out, shovel away, and wait for the sunshine. *I'll let my husband and son take care of that, as I'm not even quite capable of laundry.* Just as everyone strives to clear every inch of blizzard snow in anticipation of spring, I will take a deep breath, stay properly focused, and strive for calm. Soon the snow will be gone, and I will be one snowfall closer to the end of my cancer journey. I suspect at the end of my treatments I will be the crazy-ass patient to request every test, scan, and procedure available to make sure the cancer is gone...not a single trace in my body. The doctor will tell me it isn't medically necessary, and I will have to trust her and lean on my faith. As I look outdoors at the pure white miracle of God's creation, I realize that just like the weathermen can't always accurately predict, neither can the doctors. It is a time when I must accept a quote I embraced so many months ago, "*Let your faith be bigger than your fear.*"

The wisdom in this story: Someone told me recently that after cancer you have to accept your new normal. I pray this isn't my new normal—the always waiting, wondering when the next cell might appear. I'd rather have snowflakes.

The Shower

Monday, January 25

Yesterday's sadness has subsided slightly, and the plan of a warm morning shower made me smile. Delighted to have the energy to leave my bed, I shampooed the hair I no longer have and made one leg shaving cream ready before I remembered I haven't needed to shave in weeks. I shaved my legs anyway. As the warm water soothed my aches, it felt heavenly, but the steam added to my light-headedness and I kept my shower time short. While I still find most fragrances nauseating, the mild soap of my childhood and my favorite moisturizing cream made today feel like a spa day.

The wisdom in this story: Never, ever take anything for granted — even the ability to follow your regular morning shower routine.

Just Be There

Wednesday, January 27

The weather has cooperated enough for the kids to go back to school, but I am at home for another sick day. It seems that it takes me almost a full week to recover from a round of chemo. For today anyway, I am still certainly not well enough to be a teacher of six-year-olds. I was seldom sick as a kid, but I recall my missed school days well, and they were good days. Being at home sick meant crawling into my parents' empty king-sized bed. A bedroom television in those days was a luxury, and they had one. While the only show I remember watching while home sick was *The Price is Right*, I do remember so much more about those days. I remember the cool washcloth mom so gently placed on my forehead, the fuzzy towel so carefully tucked beside me in case of emergency *(no cold ugly vomit buckets in that house)*, and the presence of someone who loved me more than life itself. Mom knew how to just *be there*. She drifted in and out of the room with deliveries of cinnamon sugar toast, chicken noodle soup, crackers, and jello. Jello in the '70s wasn't the snack-pack tear off the lid type...it took time, love, and care *or at least boiled water* to prepare. In my eight-year-old mind, jello meant someone loved you. I remember never having to ask for anything. Mom waited on me patiently, and had a way of just showing up at the moment I felt I was needing something. Forty years later, my husband and children have stepped into this role as I recover from chemo. There have been cool washcloths, fuzzy towels, cinnamon sugar toast, chicken noodle soup, crackers, and Italian ice *(sadly, I can't seem to tolerate jello, yet then again I've only tried the snack-pack type)*. While they do an incredible job taking care of me, I sometimes have to *ask* for things, which *makes me feel helpless*. My mom just knew. Sometimes the asking comes in the form of catching someone as they walk past me at just the right moment. Sometimes I yell loudly over their electronics to get their attention. And sometimes, I resort to more modern ways and actually text them, within the walls of our home, my list of requests. *And every single time, I feel helpless.* They don't mind helping, and always try to be sure they bring exactly what I need. I recently asked my oldest daughter to bring me a small bottle of water. We were out of *small* bottles, so she brought me a *large* bottle and also a small cup full of water. As she cautiously said, "I didn't know which you would want," I felt *awful.* This poor child had actually spent a moment fretting over how to adequately satisfy my need. Teenagers shouldn't have to do that. In fact, *no one* should have to do that, and so I will share. Someone recently asked me how to best help a newly diagnosed cancer patient. I sent her a list of helpful tips and ideas of things that had brought comfort to me. What I should have said is, "*Just be there.*" Throughout this cancer journey, I have discovered that there are three ways people respond to a patient's needs in these type situations:

1. There are the people who tell you they will do anything in the world for you. They insist that you call them if you need a thing, *(which of course means you have to ask).* Most patients don't like to ask.

2. There are the people who offer you a list of ways they can help. While similar to #1, the choices seem to make a patient feel a bit less needy. My best example of this was shortly after my first surgery. A dear friend texted to say, "*I'm free today. I'll come cook for you, I'll clean for you, I'll just sit with you. Tell me what you need.*" I needed to get out of the house. I asked her to pick me up and take me to lunch. Best day ever.

3. Then, there are the people who just know how to be there. They shuffle about their own lives without ever forgetting to remind you that they are there. Just as mom drifted in and out of the room with deliveries of cinnamon sugar toast, chicken

noodle soup, crackers, and jello; they drift in and out of your lives with heartfelt cards, meals on the doorstep, and offers of prayer. Sometimes they even bring smoothies, *(way better than jello)*. They show up, without being intrusive, sometimes without even being seen. They find ways both big and small to let you know they care. Their presence warms one's heart in a way that only a mom can do, and helps a family to feel deeply loved.

While we have appreciated every single way loved ones have reached out to us during this most difficult time, and are humbled by your love, it is still hard to ask for help. For those who recognized a need without making us feel needy or helpless, we are grateful. *I am fighting the hardest battle I have ever known.*

The wisdom in this story is a thought-provoking quote from a breast cancer survivor named Debra in "What Got Me Through" (American Cancer Society): "My advice is to remember that only you can fight your cancer. Other people can do the laundry, make meals, and even wipe away tears. You must — even if it's the first time in your life — think of yourself first. No one can fight this battle as well as you can."

What's Next

Thursday, January 28

According to Wikipedia, "*I'm Going to Disney World!* is an advertising campaign slogan, used in a series of television commercials by the Walt Disney Company that began airing in 1987. Used to promote the company's theme park resort, the commercials are most often broadcast following the Super Bowl and feature an NFL player shouting the phrase while celebrating the team's victory immediately after the championship game. These commercials have also promoted champions from other sports, and winners of non-sport competitions. Disney refers to the campaign as "*What's Next*" in reference to the commercial's usual format, which has the star appear to be answering a question posed by an unseen narrator — *"What are you going to do next?"* after his or her moment of triumph. Most ads feature the song *When You Wish Upon a Star* and end with a shot of fireworks over Cinderella's Castle. So here goes:

Setting: A Loving Home

To Be Broadcast: After Chemotherapy #3

The Star: Michele B

Moment of Triumph: Body Returning to Normalcy after Treatment

Team's Victory: One Step Closer to Cancer-Free

Script:
Unseen Narrator: So, Michele. What are you going to do next?
Michele: I'm going to Disney World!

The family celebrates after these words, and an airline is booked. *When You Wish Upon a Star* echoes throughout Michele's mind and she can finally envision a shot of fireworks over Cinderella's Castle. Fade to black. Is this real? It isn't a dream. It isn't a television commercial. My flight is booked. Provided there are no unforseen medical emergencies in the next week, my son and I will be flying to Florida to join my husband and the girls for Cheer Nationals. My head is spinning, and not from the chemo. This is truly a dream realized. It is so very important for me to be there, and to be honest, I wasn't sure it could happen. I need to find my way out of the bathroom today, and find some foods I can tolerate that will help give me the strength I need to travel. Booking this flight was a monumental step in my healing. One more way of saying "*I can do it.*" Some Florida sunshine might be just what I need, and will help me prepare for my final round of chemotherapy and the 33 rounds of radiation to follow.

The wisdom in this story: "Dreams really do come true." (Disney)

The Cheer Bow

Saturday, January 30

Today was the girls' State Finals Cheerleading Championship *(not to be confused with Nationals to be held soon in Disney)*. I was informed last evening that the senior mothers decided it would be fun to show spirit by wearing cheer bows in their hair to today's competition. As a mother explained the idea to me, and I was so very obviously reminded *I have no hair*, I was almost speechless. *No, I was mad.* How could this group of moms be so inconsiderate to choose a hair bow for the mothers of seniors to wear. In the past it was a special t-shirt, a hat, *(oh my – hats would have been appropriate this year)* but no, a hair bow – a big, sparkly, glittery cheer bow. The *"normal me"* would absolutely despise even the thought of wearing a cheer bow, but the *"cancer me"* suddenly felt left out. While I had already felt a little isolated this year, this was just too much to handle. It wasn't about the bow, or even the reminder that I have no hair, but it was about the realization that once again I can't *just be mom...*mom in every sense of the word, even if it means plopping a big chunky cheer bow on top of my head. I had just unexpectedly spent my entire afternoon at the oncologist's office receiving fluids, stomach meds, and steroids. It was a combination of goodies to help me even just function after a lousy, slow week recovering from chemo. It was a tearful, frustrating day and emotions were already running high. So the talk about the cheer bows wasn't what I needed at that moment. I spouted out some ugly, yet truthful words and told the mom that it wasn't really important for me to fit in with them. I went to bed sad. I felt like I was 12 years old. I actually lost sleep over the hair bow thing, feeling the need to apologize to someone. I realized that cancer sometimes makes me sensitive about literally everything...*even cheer bows.* And then this morning came. I encountered one mom in the restroom as her daughter enveloped her in a massive, never-ending squirt of hairspray to hold mom's bow in place *(remember fragrances make me nauseous)*. As I left the restroom I asked my husband if he had seen them exit. He *(and remember he's the nice one)* rolled his eyes. I watched another girl struggle to fix a bow that had been placed in her mom's curly hair. The bow didn't want to cooperate. I watched another duo of moms giggle together like schoolgirls with bows bouncing on top of their heads. As I touched the soft knit cap on top of my bald head, I realized I didn't want to be them. It became more evident when one girl approached her mom and said, *"Mother, I really do wish you would take that stupid bow off the top of your head!"* Bless the mouth of the babe who had the guts to say it—they looked ridiculous. While it was clearly a well-intended effort to show team spirit, and they appeared to be quite proud of themselves, they looked like a bunch of menopausal crazies. I started to hear other girls approach their moms. It seemed as if some of the girls were actually embarrassed. Imagine that. I have spent the last bald-headed month of my life trying not to embarrass my children by my choice of head covering, and here these mothers were glowing with giddiness. As I sat there, happy I had no bow, but still a little melancholy about the left out feeling, it happened. A mom whose cheer daughter graduated two years ago with my son approached me. Ironically, that was the Senior Mom *"hat year."* She handed me a gift in a beautiful, pink bag. It was a hat of perhaps the softest texture I have ever felt, with a leather embossed patch stating *Love Your Melon*. She said that her sweet daughter had suggested the gift, and asked me to carefully read the gift card.

According to the card:
"Love Your Melon is an apparel brand run by college students across the country on a mission to give a hat to every child battling cancer in America. Love Your Melon has reserved more than 45,000 hats to donate to children battling cancer in the United States through its original buy one, give one program. This is equal to the

number of children currently undergoing cancer treatment in the country. The hats are donated in person at hospitals nationally by Love Your Melon college ambassadors."

The hat mom told me that hats sell out quickly and are often unavailable. My special hat took a long time to be delivered. The credit for my hat was given to a nearby university, (my alma mater and my daughter's chosen college). *I tried hard not to cry.* She told me to read the leather tag again. It took me two readings of the tag to comprehend. Love your *melon.* My *bald head* is my *melon.* I get it. And I love my melon. My melon stands for courage for all that I have endured. My melon has shown spirit each time my tired old chemo-wrecked body feels like it can't take another step out the door to be a mom. My melon, while now bare, will someday again sprout the beautiful locks that I loved to brush each evening. And my melon today, did not disgrace my dignity as a big, sparkly, glittery cheer bow may have done had I worn one. As the *"bow moms"* gathered to take a group photo, I actually hoped for a moment that someone would ask me to be included. I even whispered to my husband that I wanted to be included. He asked why. I giggled when I answered, *"Because I'd be the only one that looks normal."* I wasn't included. But that's okay. It truly isn't important for me to fit in with them. I think I'm really more of a hat mom anyway, and the hat mom who reached out to me today has touched my heart deeply.

This wisdom in this story: Why fit in, when you were born to stand out?

AND THE DISCLAIMER: If you happen to be a "cheer bow mom" who is reading this, please do not be offended. Someone told me recently "a cancer patient is the person in the center ring and can say anything she wants to anyone, anywhere. She can complain and whine and moan and curse the heavens and say, 'Life is unfair' and 'Why me?' That's the payoff for being in the center ring. No apologies needed." (Susan Silk and Barry Goldman.)

Smile Again

Tuesday, February 2

My story, *The Cheer Bow*, sure did generate a lot of emotion. Many sent messages and sweet texts to me — your words were heartwarming and overwhelming. Surprising, yet not, I haven't heard a word from any *"bow moms"* even though some claim to read my stories regularly. I was deeply hurt about the incident, but if you recall the details of my first story, it wasn't about the bow insomuch as it was just another reminder that I can't *simply be mom.* I don't think for one moment that there was an ill-intentioned effort to *exclude* me. These moms just weren't thinking to *include* me, and that is the part that hurt the most. It's easy for people to say that they never stop thinking about you and that you are always in their thoughts and prayers, but to show it is something completely different. They weren't thinking about me, but they were thinking about themselves and I suppose I could stretch it to say their daughters *(boy did that backfire for some).* But when someone close in your life, deep in your heart is struggling, it takes more than just living your life as usual to be a good friend. It requires you to think about them — a lot. It actually requires you to mean what you say and never stop thinking about them. It requires you to think about how your words, actions, and deeds may make them feel — *every single day.* Suffice it to say, you know they would do the same for you. So I'll close with this: "Don't ever assume my stories are about you, but if you are affected, you probably have something to feel guilty about. Taking offense where none is offered should initiate some self-reflection." *(unknown).* It's a little sad to me that sometimes in life, people would rather ignore you than admit they were wrong.

The wisdom in this story: "It's not about who hurt you and

broke you down. It's about who was always there and made you smile again." (unknown)

The Cancer Basket

Wednesday, February 3

There was a story my parents loved to tell about the time my father served in Vietnam. While he was away, my mother never balanced the checkbook — *not once*. As the mother of an infant and toddler, she was quite busy. She lived with her sister, and in exchange for being able stay there, cleaned her sister's house — to her sister's *very meticulous* standards. My mom took me to a children's hospital regularly, where doctors cared for my hip *(developmental dysplasia)*. I was the infant who got car sick on the hour-long trip, so even that was an adventure. While I can't recall them saying how long Dad's tour of duty lasted, Mom always said that she felt hers lasted longer. This made them both laugh. But, back to the checkbook — In my father's absence my mother monitored her spending carefully, kept papers tidy, and put everything neatly in a shoebox. When dad finally came home, he balanced the checkbook. Mom's totals were off, and while I can't remember the exact amount, it was mere *pennies*. Something tells me the amount may have been a dime, but I wouldn't want to over-exaggerate the error. While I always loved the shoebox story, I'm much more of a basket kind of girl... hand-woven baskets, plastic baskets, even laundry baskets to help keep my life organized. After my first surgery, one of my dearest friends brought me a "comfort basket" full of all of the things her family loved best. I was a magnet to the homemade cookies, but the huge assortment of other special things she had so carefully selected soon became my family's favorite things, too. And there was the basket — gorgeous, brown with handles, and big — *really, really big*. Somehow that basket found a special spot in my kitchen and became the *cancer basket*. It was at first a nice place to store literature, but as the weeks post-diagnosis turned into months, it became the place where I put anything cancer related that I didn't feel like dealing with at the moment. Cross-checking insurance paperwork with medical bills is time consuming; comprehending biopsy results, test results, and medical reports daunting; filing admissions and discharge papers cumbersome; and reading *What Side Effects to Expect* and *When to Call the Oncologist* information sheets downright depressing. So into the basket these things went. And then there was the pay, *or lack of.* I used my last available sick day in November. While I am fortunate to have partial pay disability coverage, it is in this type of situation, never quite enough. We manage to pay our bills, but it's all a little scary. While I'm usually pretty precise in knowing exactly what funds we have available, and where every penny of our paychecks go, intermittent work and partial pay makes things complicated. Days I work I get district pay, days I don't it's partial through our disability insurance. I glance at the amounts, send my husband to the bank with checks to deposit, and toss all of the pay stubs into the basket. This is most definitely not the ideal way to manage household finance, but nothing about this journey has been ideal. Now on the school district end of things, everyone is efficient *(and compassionate)*. Since I'm a leave-without-pay employee, my dear principal has to approve every single absence before the system will allow a substitute teacher request. She does so promptly, even when said request comes in a frantic text from me in my bed at the ER, or on a Sunday afternoon when I decide that losing my voice may affect my ability to teach. And she *never* makes me feel as if I am bothersome. My school secretary is responsible for handling my substitute teacher requests, doctor excuses, and my hourly time sheets. She does it all with the most incredible patience and bright smile. Our benefits-coordinator in the administrative office deals regularly with my short-term *(now long-term)* disability paperwork and the reports submitted by my many doctors. Every time I try to thank her she says, "I'm just doing my job." Then there is me, a lot like my mom during a time of crisis, and I have ignored the papers that need my attention. Just like my mom, I have monitored my spending carefully, kept my papers tidy, and put everything neatly *(okay, maybe not so neatly)*, in the cancer basket. While I still need to take the time to sort, organize, and file all that the basket holds, I know what is in there. I know that where the district pay stub looks lacking, a partial pay might soften the hurt a bit. While I know my estimates of what we have may be off, and I know it's by much more than a dime, there is enough to keep on keeping on. And I know there is enough to do Disney. I made the full payment just yesterday. My amazing school secretary sent my bank card number to Mickey.

The wisdom in this story: Sometimes in a moment of crisis, it is really okay to put everything neatly in a shoebox.

Southwest

Friday, February 5

Southwest Airlines with my son.

The wisdom in this story: Sunny skies ahead.

Growing Older

Saturday, February 6

Happy Birthday to ME!
Yes, I'm wearing Mickey Mouse ears.

The wisdom in this story: "Do not regret growing older. It is a privilege denied to many." (unknown)

No Bad Hair Days

Sunday, February 7

There comes a time when comfort is more important than appearance. My scalp has been sweaty at the sports venues and in the rush to get from place to place. Without even a thought--off came the bandeau from my head, and if I say so myself *I'm rockin' the baldness*. It's funny, because I don't really care. I am here and that's what matters—and better yet, no bad hair days for me.

The wisdom in this story: Beauty is on the inside.

Family Day

Monday, February 8

Today is our last full day in Disney. The cheerleading coaches designated today as Family Day, which means the team will split and the girls can visit parks as they choose with their own families. It is a gift that I hadn't realized was part of the cheerleading schedule. I will treasure this day with my family. The kids want to do it all, which reminds me of our first Disney trip with strollers. The parks seemed overwhelming to me; the strollers heavy to push; and yet somehow my family and I *(along with my sister and her three young children)*, managed to visit every park and do everything we had hoped to do while there. We were exhausted but happy, and quite proud of ourselves. While every park in one day for today sounds a little unrealistic; I have teenagers instead of toddlers, and the stroller has been replaced with a motorized Wheelie Car for me, *(I can't bring myself to calling it a wheelchair)*. It will be a great day and "last hurrah" before Thursday's chemo. My cancer journey is in a way, a little like a theme park visit. The surgeries, procedures, and treatments seemed overwhelming to me, the sickness hard to bear, and yet somehow, my medical team and I will soon have accomplished everything that is needed for me to be cured. We will be exhausted but happy, and quite proud of ourselves. But for today, I need to stay properly focused and toss cancer aside. Today is Family Day in *"The Happiest Place on Earth" (Disney)*.

The wisdom in this story: An adventure awaits me.

Dream Builders

Tuesday, February 9

I have always loved quotes, and the Dream Builder quotes from Walt Disney himself posted around Animal Kingdom made me smile. In his words:

"Togetherness. To me, means teamwork."

"Whatever we accomplish belongs to our entire group, a tribute to our combined effort."

"It's kind of fun to do the impossible."

In my own words, these past four days of togetherness have meant the world to me. My daughters embraced my public baldness, crippled-ness, and struggle to keep up without ever hinting at any embarrassment; my husband and son met my every need with Wheelie Car transport and much-needed strong arms to grab; family and friends alike dried my occasional tears — many happy tears, and some, well, just *cancer sucks* tears. Their love and affection was a display of teamwork that made this trip possible. I can proudly say, "I did it!" because of their combined effort. Ten short days ago, I made an unexpected trip to the oncologist's office for fluids, steroids, and stomach meds. I struggled through the weekend and ended up at Urgent Care. An antibiotic, more steroids, and a cough medicine to help me sleep followed, and yet I remained doubtful about the trip. Even at the airport, I wasn't sure I had made the right decision. I was feeling hopeless and the trip seemed impossible. But I hopped on that plane, and I did it! *It wasn't easy, but I did it.* To be perfectly honest, there were parts of the trip that were a real struggle, both physically and emotionally. But Walt says it best:

The wisdom in this story: "It's kind of fun to do the impossible." (Walt Disney)

146

Last Chemo

Thursday, February 11

TODAY IS MY LAST CHEMO. I've accepted the fact that
chemo kicks me in the ass, and simply plan to spend the next
full week on the couch, in the bathroom, and in my bed. My
family will again live life to the fullest, and I'll be the
bystander, watching it all happen in a blur. I hate these weeks,
but with each step of fighting cancer, I am able to look back
and say, "*I did it.*" I will be one step closer to being cured.
Radiation will begin for me in early March, and once again the
fear of the unknown will terrify me. I've been told I'll be tired
but not sick, and that my skin will be tender, perhaps raw. My
sister's advice of one day at a time will keep me going and my
dear friend's advice to stay properly focused will help my
mind from wandering too much. The promise of jelly donut
celebrations at the end *(when jelly donuts will taste good again),*
and a whole bag of Oreos from a friend who checks in
regularly await me. My breakfast and lunch friends eagerly
await the return of our mom sanity breaks. We have a lot of
catching up to do, and the word cancer will be banned from
our conversations. We will sit in the booth for hours talking
about our kids, and we will tip our server generously. It will
feel so good to return to life without treatments. But I'm not
there yet. There are still some difficult months ahead. I'll
have 33 Radiation treatments *(daily for seven weeks),* more tests
and scans, and the eventual removal of my medi-port. There
are days I will feel incredibly defeated, and other days I will
feel like I've accomplished the impossible. That is the reality of
being a cancer patient. May God richly bless those of you who
read my stories regularly, pray for me daily, and reach out to
simply hold my hand. While *"I couldn't have done it without
you"* sounds so cliché, it is so very true. Never again will I
underestimate the seriousness of a Stage 1 diagnosis and

I hope that others don't either. While I'm feeling thankful that my cancer wasn't found in lymph nodes, and so very blessed that I will be cured, Stage 1 has been my awful...my very own personal kind of hell, and there's no nice way to say it. But as the song goes, "I've still got a lot of fight left in me." *(Rachel Platten)*.

The wisdom in this story: It always seems impossible until it is done.

Be Mine

Sunday, February 14

Thursday, Friday, and Saturday passed with uncomfortableness but minimal side effects, and I should have known it was too good to be true. I was elated. I spent time enjoying family, thinking that perhaps my body had hardened to the harshness of chemo and was going to survive round #4 without incident. On Sunday morning, my husband surprised me with a jelly donut and some beautiful roses. *Damn those jelly donuts.* The morning was okay, but by afternoon my chemo sweats and muscle aches had intensified. Nausea and stomach issues returned. Fatigue was the worst it had ever been. As usual, I went from couch to bed and back again. My kids seemed to notice my absence on this day dedicated to showing love to one another, and each took a random turn here and there passing quietly through my room to tell or ask me something. I rested but didn't sleep. While I longed to be active, I relished in the quiet. Late afternoon, my Valentine of almost 30 years passed through the room. He seemed afraid that his presence would wake me, and cautiously came to the edge of the bed. My tears came from nowhere, and I told him for probably the millionth time how much I hate all of this cancer stuff. He held my hand gently while I told him I'm tired. I don't feel like a fighter. I swore that if cancer ever returned I'd never tell a soul, I'd just let it grow until I am gone. I know. I sound pathetic. *I feel pathetic.* I've said it before and I'll say it again, this is my hell. This is much, much, harder than I had ever, ever imagined. It goes far beyond the physical discomfort and reaction to the harsh drugs that flow into my body every 21 days. It goes far beyond my physical appearance of scars, swelling, and hair loss. It goes deep into the heart of what makes us whole...*emotion.* And it's hard. I'm not the wife I want to be. I'm not the mother I want to be. I'm not the sister, friend, or teacher I want to be. I feel like I am just here, and since my diagnosis I have functioned through the days almost thoughtlessly. Life has been nothing but a blur. We talked for awhile, and I finally found the word that helped me to understand today's sadness. Radiation. Not really the radiation, but once again the fear of the unknown. While I should be celebrating the end of chemo, I am already anxious about the radiation that will soon follow. I hadn't slept well the night before, and was awake about every hour reading everything there is to know about radiation. *Never search online.* The tears flowed longer than I'd like to admit with my husband at my side. I apologized, and he looked helpless. He stayed long enough to provide comfort, but not so long to allow me to delve deeper into my self-pity. I had let my fear grow bigger than my faith, and it momentarily took over. I'm afraid, and I know this scares him, too. But he is mine, along with the three incredible children I feel blessed to love on this Valentine's Day. They will help me fight until I feel whole again...someday able to be the wife, mother, sister, friend, and teacher I long to be. The house is quiet, my husband now softly snoring beside me. *(Much louder usually deserves a nudge or a yell, sometimes even a kick.)* Yes, even through sadness, I maintain my sense of humor. I will fall asleep soon, after lots of prayer. I need to refocus and remember that I can do this...*all of it*...no matter how defeated I may sometimes feel. There will be a happily-ever-after to my story — getting there just sort of sucks sometimes.

The wisdom in this story: I am blessed to have a wonderful husband and three incredible children to love on this Valentine's Day. And the best part...even on my darkest days, they never seem to stop loving me back.

Sick and Tired of Being Sick and Tired

Monday, February 15

I have been sick for over a month. Not cancer sick, not chemo sick, just winter cold, cough, and ache sick. I was coughing at my January chemo appointment. At Disney in early February, I was finding myself unusually short of breath. Even with steroids, I lost my voice completely for almost three weeks, frustrating to me, *but to be honest I think my family liked it.* I still can't speak much above a whisper. The oncologist's office called it viral, urgent care gave me three prescriptions, and yet here I sit with a mucous mess lingering somewhere between my bronchial and my lungs. A single cough can make my already weak and tired body feel drained. I just want to feel better and have one night of uninterrupted sleep. But my blood counts look beautiful. *Thank heavens my blood counts look beautiful.* The doctor laughed a little when I told her that was my reward for spending 26 years in first grade. The final round of chemo was my choice. The doctor said I seemed sick enough to warrant delaying it, but my strong numbers gave her confidence that it was also okay to proceed. Me, I want to be done—*as soon as possible.* So now I battle round #4 side effects while adding some nasty over-the-counter medications to my already upset stomach. Again, I find myself crying. I worry about myself sometimes, but I have enough good days to know that I'm okay. I'm just not a very patient patient, which I have known since day one. I talked with someone recently who has a relative going through chemo treatments. This person told me that the patient was doing well because they kept busy and didn't sit around dwelling on their cancer. I immediately felt defensive. I explained that I don't dwell on my cancer either. I work as often as I feel able, and try incredibly hard to never let anything interfere with my efforts to be a good mom, including having my teenage son practically drag me through the airport to get me to Disney and swallowing my pride when I first climbed aboard the handicapped wheelie cars in the theme parks. I explained that I try hard not to wear my heart on my sleeve, but that some days are harder than others and cancer is something I'm struggling to endure. This person told me that she guessed some people have to be that way, to complain to help them get through it. *I guess that was a polite way of putting me in a category of people who complain.* Then I sit silently and listen — I sit and listen to some of these same healthy people complain that they're so tired. Their lives are hard. That was me once, but cancer has changed things. While cancer doesn't stop me from complaining about my winter cold, cough, and ache sick, I know there is a bigger picture — the bigger battle — *the hardest fight I've ever known.* For all that I have endured and all that is to come, I think I've earned forgiveness for those occasional heart-on-my-sleeve moments. My world of cancer is one that should allow me to freely feel however I may feel, without ever having to feel the need to explain myself. Sometimes when I'm sick and tired of being sick and tired, frustrated that I cannot function in a way to which I am accustomed, I crumble. I complain. But I don't think I ever *dwell,* and I become defensive toward the people who make me feel as if I do. So, last night...I couldn't sleep again. I didn't want to search radiation. I searched quotes. I love quotes. I found one that made me laugh out loud. I'll leave it as today's wisdom:

The wisdom in this story: "No, I don't need therapy. I just need people to stop pissing me off." (unknown)

The Wicker

Saturday, February 20

When I was a child, my father worked tirelessly to build a beautiful screened-in porch. It became the best feature of an already lovely house. My mother spent way too much money on a gorgeous set of white wicker furniture, but through the years she got every penny's worth. During my teenage years, and for many years afterward, that's where you would find her. Late at night when I arrived home from an evening with friends, my job waitressing, or late-nights at school early in my teaching career, we would sit together on the wicker and talk—*for hours.* That wicker was there for us through happy days and heartaches. We shared laughter and shed tears during wedding planning and my infertility that followed. That wicker was the furniture where her grandchildren ate Popsicles in summer months and she calmed my insecurities about being a good mom. While I don't remember her replacing the wicker, I know it became mine sometime before she died, as it was on the screened-in porch of my first home. When we built our new home, the home-design lended itself greatly to not one beautiful porch, but three. Our screened-in porch is the place for an outdoor dining area, the porch off of our sunroom/master bedroom a quiet respite with beautiful view of the mountain, and the front porch—well, that was the place for mom's wicker—a view of the action of the whole farm, and so pretty and welcoming for all who rang the front doorbell (*guests to the front door usually have to walk past a sidewalk of dog poop, so the attractiveness of the porch helps a bit.*). While we are delighted to have three porches, it is sad that our lives are so hectic that they are seldom used. We aren't typically home long enough to sit on a porch. Even so, years and weather take its toll on everything, and last Spring, the wicker was looking pretty irreparable, even beginning to

153

rot in spots. It had seen its better days. I told my husband I couldn't bear to put mom's wicker out for the trash, and instructed him to someday have a little bonfire when I wasn't home. He and my son seemed to agree that it had a little life left in it for an area in the basement. *I think they were sad to see it go, too.* I replaced the wicker with two white rocking chairs, *Happy Mother's Day, Mom*. I demanded to the family that we were going to use them. I think we did — twice. Then I became the mom who went from never sitting still, to doing nothing but rotating from bed to couch, to bed again. During this last round of chemo, I've been mostly in bed. My middle child, my high school senior, does the best job finding me. It is here in my bed that we have giggled about boys; cried tears about friends *(sometimes when you are a teenager and your mom has cancer you find out who your true friends really are);* planned dairy princess events; talked about college scholarships; looked at prom gowns; and shared conversations about dorm-styles and prospective college roommates. While I hate that I'm in bed for much of this, I have been still and fully focused on her words. She has my undivided attention until I sometimes catch myself dozing and she smiles lovingly and gently says goodnight. My husband and I have raised such a lovely, caring, confident daughter. Things are falling into place nicely for her. She has an incredibly bright future ahead of her, and these last months before her graduation will pass quickly. I know that, and I think she knows that. Yesterday, I started on a new antibiotic from my wonderful family doctor; and visited my oncologist for an infusion of fluids, steroids, nausea meds, and potassium *(lacking from being unable to eat)*. I pray that the combination of all of these things pull together quickly for me, as a full six weeks of being sick is just too much. The snow has melted a bit and I'll have some porch sitting in my future. While I have three porches from which to choose, I might need my strong son to bring up a special, tired old wicker chair from the basement.

The wisdom in this story: Hanging out with your grown-up kids is like visiting with the best parts of yourself.

The Mall

Monday, February 22

Today would have been my mother's 81st birthday. Cancer took her at age 66. She never lived long enough to grow old. While I wonder what my mom may have looked like at the age of 81, I cannot picture her old. To me, she will be forever young. Gray hair only at the temples, beautiful flawless skin, always a great lipstick, and youthful in so many ways — it is truly a blessing to remember her young and before cancer. My mother had a laugh that could bring you to tears, and loved almost everything about being a mom. *She didn't love the mall.* The mall was too much walking for my mom, and there were never enough benches. Yet, I asked, and she took me. Many of my memories include our shopping adventures. As an adult, I now hate the mall. The mall is too much walking for me, and there are never enough benches. Yet, my girls ask, and I take them. My oldest daughter and I recently had a conversation about her *"things to do before college"* list, with a laptop purchase being high priority on the list. We are an Apple household, so the purchase of a laptop would mean a trip to the Apple Store — *at the mall.* For those who have been following my stories, my life lately hasn't included the mall. It's mostly couch, bed, couch, with the occasional Disney wheelie car thrown in for good measure. For the past six weeks I have been coughing. I haven't felt well. Where the congestion/cold/cough didn't kick me, the chemo did. Finally, on Friday I started an antibiotic that I should have received six weeks ago, but that's another whole story in itself. The antibiotic, combined with some replenishing drugs in my port helped rejuvenate my whole system; the only thing still lacking, a voice with which to teach first graders, granting me freedom to return to work and feel normal. However, my own children have grown accustomed to hearing me only whisper, and on Sunday morning I seemed like perfectly normal mom. *And she asked.* The child who has tended to my every need since diagnosis, who has loved and cared deeply asked, "So, if you're feeling better, would today be a good day to get my laptop?" I silently sighed. The *mall.* I did what any other good antibiotic-filled mom would do, and answered, "Sure!" I was feeling good, maybe not *mall good,* but *mom good* and ready for adventure. Sunday morning, light crowds, and my daughter's first laptop *(when many of her friends have owned one all of high school).* Our trip to the Apple Store went as things usually do at the Apple Store...*flawlessly.* In my opinion, the whole world would be a better place if run like an Apple Store. I suggested a quick stop in the Vera Bradley store to purchase a laptop bag to protect this huge new investment. I told my daughters I'd be on the bench while they shopped, but they reminded me of the beauty of the Vera Bradley store — chairs — *two gorgeous resting chairs for tired moms.* I joined my daughters in the store. I sat my bald-headed self down on a chair and smiled. We were shopping. *At the mall.* Shopping for college. I felt a tear trickle down my cheek, along with the kind of cough that even the best antibiotics can't cure. A lovely sales girl offered me a bottle of water, and not out of pity, but out of genuine kindness. I accepted. I wondered for a moment how pathetic I must have looked, but remembered that I had applied the lipstick that others say does wonders for my tired face. My daughter found a laptop bag quickly, and was then drawn to a sale area. She is the kid who loves a bargain and always buys her backpacks off-season. She brought one over and asked if I thought it matched the purple laptop bag she had selected. The sparkle in her eyes told me she loved it and I said it was perfect. The sales girl's question that followed left me almost speechless. "Did you know that's our *Breast Cancer Awareness* pattern?" My daughter looked at me, and our eyes locked momentarily before I had to look away. I didn't even know Vera Bradley had a special line, and it didn't appear that my daughter did either. I quietly whispered, "*I have breast cancer.*" The sales girl smiled knowingly as if she had already guessed. We learned that Vera Bradley's primary corporate cause is breast cancer research. The company is dedicated to eradicating breast cancer as a life-threatening disease. When it came time to pay, the kindness continued. The sales girl slipped a fluffy velour breast cancer pattern blanket into our bag and said, "This is our store's gift to you." It felt really awkward having an expensive item for which I didn't pay placed into my bag, but I accepted. I tried really hard not to cry. We hugged. She went on to tell briefly about her neighbor who had breast cancer. "I slipped one of these blankets on her porch, *you know*—just as a way of reaching out." I did know. Cancer touches too many lives. It takes too many. As much as I hate the mall, I am blessed to have been able to spend this day with my daughters, our day deeply touched by the kindness of a sales girl whose path crossed ours only briefly. I hope that my daughters never have to wonder what I'll look like at the age of 81. I pray I will be here to show them. I'm fighting this awful disease so that I can have many, many more birthdays. I hope to be 101. I'll be the one driving the wheelie car in the mall...the old lady with the great lipstick whose laughter can bring you to tears.

The wisdom in this story: My mom never allowed us to buy her a present—she always preferred to buy for us. Happy Birthday, Mom. I think you sent the blanket from Heaven. While I think it was meant for me, it looks just perfect for a college dorm...

The Port

Wednesday, February 24

I've never been thrilled to have a medi-port. One was strongly suggested due to my crappy veins and the strength of my chemo drugs. It was explained that if they missed a vein during regular IV infusion, I could suffer from chemo burns and tissue damage. That alone was enough to convince me to get a port…but I've hated the port. The procedure wasn't easy, the healing of the incision imperfect enough to cause concern about infection, and it's just something inside of me that doesn't belong. Now, while in many ways it truly has been an *easy button* of sorts, easier than multiple attempts to draw blood or infuse chemo properly, I can't wait to have it removed. At my last chemo, I was told the port would need to be flushed every four to six weeks when not in use.

Me: "When not in use? Will they need it during radiation?"

Nurse: "No, they won't need it."

M: "So, why can't I just get it out?"

N: (tentatively) "You can," (followed by a whisper of) "but some people like to keep them longer."

M: "How MUCH longer?"

N: (quietly) "Oh, six months or more, but it's totally your choice."

At that moment, I was tired. No more questions. I decided to rest and let the chemo drip into my port, all while wondering *"why in the world would anyone wait SIX months to get their port removed?"* It made no sense to me, or perhaps I was simply in denial. Almost two weeks have passed since that conversation. My chemo fog has lifted. While my eyes are heavy and tired, I cannot sleep. Here it is 3AM, and it just occurred to me why people wait six months to have their port removed. In six months, there will be mammograms, ultrasounds, scans. People wait because they want to make sure that...

...the cancer isn't still there.

The wisdom in this story: Sometimes middle-of-the night insomnia can be worse than an internet search.

Rested and Ready

Thursday, February 25

I am finally well enough to return to work today and although my voice is still not 100%, I am ready! I will smile with my students and celebrate with my colleagues. Returning to work means that even though the chemo knocked me down, I had the strength it took to get back up again, and again, and again, and again. I will always remember my chemotherapy time as not one, but four big challenges. Just as high school football players vividly recall plays from each quarter of the big game, I will vividly remember each of my four rounds of chemo. While on many, even most days I felt defeated, in the end I won—I am done with chemo and I feel weak but good. These next two weeks will be my off-season. I will get stronger each and every day. While it's doubtful that I will ever again feel the way I felt before diagnosis, these next two weeks will be the most normal I will have felt in a long time. Two weeks to rest and get ready for radiation.

The wisdom in this story: Resting and then ready to fight. Again.

Simulation

Friday, March 4

As defined, simulation is the imitation of the operation of a real-world process. Theme parks offer guests motion simulation thrill rides that simulate what an astronaut might experience aboard a spacecraft. I'm not exactly a thrill-seeking individual, and for many years it took a lot of courage for me to be brave enough to ride those rides. I felt nauseous and weak in the knees, but the rides were just phenomenal. I have great memories of the rides, but also recall the feeling of relief when my feet touched the ground. Nowadays, I simply admit that I'm content to sit on the bench. I have spent a lot of time on benches, couches, and in bed these last few months. While my voice is still raspy and weak, I have bounced back from the chemo in such a way that my watery eyes and lack of hair are the only observable signs that I'm still a sick person. I feel good, and I was given a full two weeks to rest and regain strength before radiation treatments begin. But first, simulation. I smiled a little when the radiation oncologist told me that I would have an appointment for simulation prior to my actual radiation treatments. *Simulation – who uses that word – apparently only theme park operators and radiation oncologists.* Today was simulation. It took a lot of courage for me to be brave enough to walk through the door of the radiation office. I was once again more than a little terrified. I met some lovely nurses and a great new doctor *(Dr. No-Bedside-Manner" who spent a maximum of two minutes with me in the fall has since retired).* Getting ready for simulation was a lot like standing in line at a theme park. You don't realize you're waiting for something scary, because they do their best to entertain you along the way. The nurses filled my mind with names of products safe to use on my tender skin, and careful demonstrations of all that would occur during treatments.

The new doctor *(with a sweet sense of humor)* reviewed the details of my diagnosis. Before I knew it they were talking about the breathing. Apparently radiation to the left breast is a little tricky, because the heart is on the left side. To offer the safest method of radiation, one must fill the lungs completely, which pushes the heart as far away from the breast/radiation area as possible. I was given a tube that resembled a snorkel and they asked if I'd ever gone snorkeling. I nodded yes, and my mind quickly wandered to snorkeling in the swimming pool as a high school student and later, in the beautiful Caribbean as a newlywed. *The swimming pool – never a big deal.* I had grown up in the pool and was great at swimming to the edge and pushing up on the wall to get out. *The Caribbean – I was more than a little terrified.* I remember I had trouble breathing properly. I spent the first half of our snorkel time trying not to hyperventilate. My husband enjoyed all the beautiful sea creatures while I floated near the boat…and then – *I got the hang of it.* I had to talk myself through the breathing, and what a sight to behold! My honeymoon was almost 23 years ago, and I can still remember the beauty of the iridescent fish in those crystal clear waters. A blip on the computer screen in the big, scary room brought me back to reality as the nurse brought the tube to my lips. I would breathe normally two deep breaths, and then take another and hold for 13 seconds. Didn't it occur to anyone to tell these people that 13 is an unlucky number? Just as I was thinking, *no big deal,* the nurse placed a clamp on my nose, smiled, and said "This is so you can't cheat." We did some practice breaths while I was still seated, and she explained the importance of the button I held in my hand. It was a call-button of sorts, but I was instructed to push it firmly and only release it when I needed assistance or a breath. While the whole concept seemed a little ass-backwards to me, *(I think of "push the button for help"),* I was determined not to release my hold on that button. The practice breathing went just fine, and I was told to lie flat on the table…face up, thank goodness, as bad

memories of the face-down MRI flooded my mind. A
beanbag type pillow was used to make a mold of my upper
body, so that the lasers beamed to the tattoos I would receive
would help to ensure exact and proper placement on the table
with each treatment. Just as the theme parks wanted to make
sure that the thrill-ride experiences felt like an actual space
flight, the oncology office wanted to make sure that my
radiation simulation felt like an actual treatment. The doctor
wished me well, waved a pretend hypnosis clock and said
"forget about chemo, the worst is over," and left the room. The
nurse reminded me that while she would be leaving the room,
she could always hear me, and to release my hold on the
button if I needed anything. The door shut, and I felt afraid. I
told myself not to hyperventilate. I had practiced. I had the
hang of it. I tried, *but without success*, to see the iridescent fish
in my mind. The breathing went okay, and while I had to talk
myself through the breathing, I didn't need to ask for
assistance. The nurse returned and told me my breathing was
great, the imaging looked good and everything was properly
prepared for radiation, except for the final step, the tattoos.
She drew on me with permanent marker. She removed the
stickers the doctor had so carefully placed. I wondered if the
tattoos would hurt, and so I asked. *I am still the patient that
always likes knowing.* She told me it would feel like a little
pinch. It was more than a pinch, and uncomfortable but not
awful. I do not foresee a real tattoo in my life — ever. When she
finished, she told me to grab her arm and she carefully helped
me rise to a seated position on the table. She told me to just sit
there for a few minutes. I felt a little nauseous and weak in the
knees. My nervousness had gotten to me. There was no
phenomenal moment like I experienced on the theme park
rides. I felt a sense of relief when my feet touched the ground.
Simulation wasn't awful, but it was scary to me. Radiation will
be scary to me. I'm still a wimpy patient. But I can do this. 33
more visits…one day at a time.

The wisdom in this story: Someday, I will return to the Caribbean. I will place a tube in my mouth and snorkel in the crystal clear waters. I will swim alongside the iridescent fish. I will hold a deep breath for 13 seconds, and I will smile.

My Cancer Angel

Wednesday, March 9

It is very hard to talk about cancer. If you talk to **someone who has never had cancer**, they just don't *get it*. While most try to be empathetic, they have no idea what you have endured both physically and emotionally. They don't recognize how different you now feel, how much your life has changed, and not necessarily in a good way. While they comment that you look good, they forget that you glance into the mirror each morning. You see a bald, swollen, older, exhausted person, only a slight glimmer of your pre-cancer-self looking back, eyes slightly diverted from the painful reflection. They don't get that their complaints about bad hair days, going to work, and even sitting in traffic seem so mundane to us, the cancer patients. We have no hair, so a bad hair day sounds appealing; we long for the normal routine of going to work; and sometimes while sitting in traffic we simply appreciate the quiet time and reflect on how lucky we are to be alive. When you talk to **someone whose loved one had cancer**, they're eager to share those stories, but don't really want to listen to yours. Usually their loved one's cancer was far worse than yours; their loved one had the best doctors and made the best medical decisions; and their loved one was never weak but always strong. **And then there are the times when you talk to the cancer patients.** Somehow, we manage to connect beautifully. There is a sisterhood in ice packs, Aquaphor, and Motrin. We are a *"no secrets"* kind of group. No question is too awkward or personal to ask. We talk about the frightening moments of diagnosis and the fear that comes with the word cancer. We talk about anesthesia, surgeries, and pain pills that we'd rather not take. We talk about medi-ports, IV drips, and all of the yucky side effects that come with chemotherapy. We talk about foods that taste awful, and rejoice when a glass of water no longer has a metallic taste.

We talk about radiation tattoos, deep inspiration breath holding, and skin care. We talk about the doctors and nurses who provide our constant care, and while we complain about every chemo drip, medicine, and side effect of said medicines, we are thankful that researchers have made these cures available to us. While we're careful not to overwhelm one another, we are smart enough to be honest, so that someone who follows a similar path can feel prepared instead of afraid. We talk about emotions, and we are accepting of one another when the tears flow. We don't try to fix it, because we know that cancer patients deserve a good cry *(and maybe a jelly donut)*. We lift each other up, and feel each other's pain when a non-cancer person says something hurtful that brings us down. I first learned about a special breast cancer patient shortly after my second surgery. I read her story in a local publication. My story mirrored hers. Detected by mammogram. No palpable lump. No family history. Lumpectomy. Re-excision. Stage 1. I wasn't sure I wanted to read further. Surely she didn't need chemo. Yes, she needed chemo followed by radiation. *Would I need chemo? Radiation?* Yes, our stories remained similar. Weeks after I read her story, in a non-cancer related way and not at my request, our paths crossed. On the phone at first, then through texting, then in the form of an *"everything you need to survive chemo"* kit she sweetly left on my front porch. This person I had never met began to follow my stories, often leaving messages of compassion, understanding, and support. I promised that someday we would meet, someday when I was well enough to go out to lunch. We met today. It should have felt awkward, but we had plenty to talk about. Lunch lasted two hours and we vowed to meet again. *I had questions – she had answers.* We shared stories, and she was someone who completely understood what I have endured both physically and emotionally. She talked about how different she now feels, and how much her life has changed. While I thought she looked fabulous, she sees only a slight glimmer of her pre-cancer self when she looks in the mirror. She said that she feels old. She is younger than me. Our lunch visit went too fast and it was hard to say goodbye to my new friend. We will have a unique future together. We will talk after each mammogram and scan, as we both pray the cancer never returns. I can't begin to adequately describe the gratitude I feel for this woman who has been by my side for months even though we didn't meet until today. When we hugged goodbye, I thanked her and the words popped out. I whispered, *"You are my angel."* I truly believe that God works in mysterious ways, and He knew I needed someone who had walked my same path to guide me. She assures me I'll do fine with radiation. Simulation was scary to her too, as were the first few radiation treatments. But then, like everything else on this cancer journey, you look back and feel a sense of accomplishment. You know that one step closer to being cured means everything. You know that while others complain about bad hair days and having to go to work, your life has deeper meaning. You will smile at the traffic and think *"no big deal"* because your life journey has been far more difficult than any day on the highway.

The wisdom in this story: Sometimes new friends are cancer angels in disguise.

Paper Chains

Wednesday, March 16

I remember making *"countdown to Christmas"* paper chains with my sister when we were kids. Construction paper links of bright reds and greens were hung neatly from the posts of our canopy beds. The idea was that one paper link was torn off each evening before bed until Santa arrived. I wasn't very good at the paper chain routine. Sometimes I would forget to tear off a link, and other times I was a bit overzealous, tearing off too many. I remember relying on my sister's always accurate count to get my own chain back to reflecting the correct number of countdown days. I have a little free time this morning before my radiation appointment, the first of 33 treatments. While I know I shouldn't be, I am nervous. Some housework desperately needs my attention, but I have another more important task on my to-do list. As juvenile as it sounds, I'm making a paper chain. I have scrapbook paper in the prettiest patterns and hues of pink all ready to be cut into strips. Glue dots make white school glue seem antique, and I will finish my project quickly. As I gently form each of the 33 links, I will say a prayer. The prayer will be simple.

Dear God,
Please heal those with cancer.
Amen

I will hang my paper chain in a prominent spot in my home for all to see. Each evening, I will tear off a link and celebrate. Thirty-three weekdays until no more cancer treatments *(if you don't count the pill I'll have to take for the next five years...).* While I won't need to rely on my sister to keep my chain accurate, I will rely on her words that have guided me throughout this entire journey...one day at a time. I can do this!

The wisdom in this story: Sometimes it's nearly impossible to lose track of the countdown days, but pretty paper chains add to the fun and anticipation.

One Down, Thirty-Two to Go

Wednesday, March 16

There isn't much to say about my first radiation treatment. There is a great deal of math and science involved in this type of treatment, which surprised me a bit. A team of physicists reviewed my plan and made some adjustments prior to today. That meant more tattoos and imaging for me, and a final approval from the doctor before we could begin. Simulation gave me a good idea what to expect, so aside from the moving machinery above me, it wasn't too awful. I even did okay with the breathing. I was on the table about a half hour due to the necessary adjustments, and was happy to leave the radiation room. As I rounded the corner to retrieve my rumpled clothing from the locker, I heard one of my two technicians cheerfully say, "I'll see you tomorrow!" Until that moment, I hadn't realized that every day really is *every* day and I'll be back doing this again in 24 short hours. My skin already feels tingly, but I assume that is all in my imagination. I feel tired, but can't really recall a time since diagnosis that I've slept well. Either way, I feel far better than I did after my first chemo treatment. And they tell me tomorrow will be even easier.

The wisdom in this story: Maybe this won't be so bad after all.

Happy Birthday to My Sister

Thursday, March 17

My uncle passed away two days before my mother's 50th birthday. It wasn't supposed to be that way. *It's never supposed to be that way.* He was going to be the one to tease her about being Over the Hill. Her birthday came and went with much sadness. Last year, my sister turned 50. I was determined to host the party of all parties. It was to be a surprise. Lime green accented with navy blue were the colors of the event for my part-Irish sister born one minute before midnight on St. Patrick's Day. Her kids had beautiful portraits taken, which would become the centerpieces. Family and friends wrote heartfelt, touching stories, which I had compiled into a scrapbook. The guest list included only her closest, most intimate friends, selected by a coworker and neighbor. My lovely sister was deserving of this special time with so many who adore her. I was only missing two details:

1. *My sister hates surprises.*
2. *My sister hates to be the center of attention.*

She became suspicious a few days before the party. She laughed at first but then threatened to not come. She asked why?!? *Why in the world would I think it was a good idea to have a party...* I told her guests why in my big nervous speech as we awaited her arrival. It was actually quite simple:

"My sister is so very worth celebrating. She is loved by all who are privileged to know her. She has raised three incredible children of her own, and has touched the lives of hundreds of others in her career as a teacher. She is a blessing to our family.

And we are alive. We are healthy. My mom's brother died just before her 50th birthday. I am alive. I am healthy. I am able to pull off an almost-surprise party for someone I love dearly." *That was last year. This year has been a little rough.* Even with the help of everyone I know, cancer would have interfered with such a party this year. But, back to last year — My sister came to the party. *Whew.* She was a bit anxious. More than a bit overwhelmed. I had selfishly put my sister out of her comfort zone in hosting a party, even though my intent was to shower her with love. Her friends appeared to have a wonderful time, but it was awkward for both of us. We exchanged very few words. While my sister wasn't upset with me, I had caused her to feel uncomfortable, embarrassed even. Weeks after the last remnants of the party were swept away, things returned to normal for us. After all, we are sisters, forever friends. While the party wasn't my best judgment and wasn't her best moment, I am so very glad that I hosted her 50th. Cancer has reminded me that not everyone reaches life's special milestones. I'm going to text my sister soon to wish her a Happy 51st Birthday. I'll text that the surprise party begins at 7PM. She won't admit it, but I know my comment will make her laugh. It will become our annual birthday joke. That alone will help erase some of the awkwardness of last year.

The wisdom in this story: "Never regret growing older. It is a privilege denied to many." (unknown)

P.S. She replied to my text.
One simple line:
"I'll be there."
Gosh, how I love her...

The Nightmare

Saturday, March 19

It's just past 3AM and I'm wide awake. They tell me radiation will make me tired. I am tired, but it's hard to discern whether I'm still chemo-tired, now radiation-tired, or simply tired because I never can seem to get an uninterrupted full night of sleep. I had my first *(and hopefully last)* radiation meltdown last night. Not meltdown in the sense of anything radioactive, but in the sense of an overwhelmed, terrified *here come the tears that won't stop* moment. As I carefully applied the special radiation lotion to my breast and surrounding area, *(disclaimer, these stories are about boobs!)*, things felt, well — different. In the area of where an underwire bra may touch *(and no, I don't wear an underwire, they are a no-no for radiation patients)*, things felt hard, tender, lumpy. My heart sank. Believe it or not, since surgery, I haven't paid a lot of attention to my boobs. One might think I'd be self-examining my breasts daily, but to be honest the scarring around my incisions make things feel lumpy anyway. But this was a different area I hadn't noticed before, and only on my surgery-side breast. I went into full-blown panic. I sat topless on the bed, seeking comfort in the form of phone calls to two "*I had radiation, too*" friends, neither whom noticed any unusual lumpiness in themselves during radiation. Always a little self-conscious and awkward, especially now, I wrapped my nearly naked self in the bedspread when my husband walked into the room. I wanted to ask the man who has been so dear to me to see if he felt what I felt, but it seems he was coming to tell me he was on his way to work. He didn't know the urgency of my concern, or the panic I was feeling. I suppose when you're a farmer, sometimes the cows don't wait; so I never asked him to check me and he just looked a little bewildered, a look that really isn't so uncommon around here post-diagnosis. I went to bed sad, mad, scared, and restless. As a child, I was a restless sleeper and dreamt a lot. The doctor told my mother that sometimes the brain of an intelligent child never stops to rest, *(don't be impressed, I lost that intelligent gene years ago and have since acquired chemo-brain)*. Yet, I truly believe that most nights my brain never stops. I dream regularly, almost every night, and I have learned that my dreams are usually an odd combination of things I have thought about during the day. Sometimes my dreams are very real, so real that I have to question myself once awake if I dreamt things or if they really happened. So, just moments ago, it wasn't a dream, it was a *nightmare*. In my dream, I was wearing one of the radiation gowns now so familiar to me, *(the shortened top-only version that ties at the waist and lets pretty much everything above all hang out)*. I was back in the mammography waiting room I haven't visited since September. A large canvas bag full of lesson plans and teachers manuals was beside me. *(I went into school from 4PM-6:30PM yesterday to get caught up, so the dream must mean I have a little school-anxiety, too!)* My radiation nurse and one technician entered the room and sort of whispered to one another, "Should we deal with her now?" In my dream, my mind was prepared for the worst— the cancer was back. There would be a need for more invasive surgeries and more chemo. I would be taking a full year off from school, *which is a nightmare in itself.* They had consulted with my surgeon. They carried a clipboard with confusing numbers all highlighted. I was prepared for the worst, but they told me the lumpiness was nothing. Good news. And then I woke up. I was sweating, not sure if it's residual chemo-sweats, menopausal-hot flashes, or the kind of sweats that come when nightmares leave you terrified. I pray my life won't always be this way, fear of everything that feels different about my body. Months ago, a dear friend told me her cancer motto was SPF—stay properly focused. I think I've lost focus. Tomorrow my bedtime routine will include a warm drink with honey, some lavender lotion on the non-radiated parts of my body, and a prayer for peace. I will ask for a nurse visit and breast exam on Monday when I go for radiation. I just hope she doesn't enter the room carrying a clipboard.

The wisdom of this story: "Nightmares exist outside of the realm of logic." (Stephen King)

Fear

Monday, March 21

I spent the better part of my weekend worrying about the area at my bra line that felt a bit unusual to me. A nurse confirmed that she also felt something. She described it as a band of muscle. I had wondered if perhaps it was muscle, ones only used recently when I maintain a hands-behind-my-head position on the radiation table. Upon further examination, the doctor was happy to diagnose the part that I described as the hardest was indeed my — wait for it — *rib*. Yes, I spent most of my weekend upset about a band of muscle and a rib that is right where it belongs. Oh, how along with these lumpy, bumpy feelings I had let my mind wander. At church yesterday, I took special note of the Pastoral Prayer. We were reminded that *He is with us with every step and every breath we take.* I thought of the breathing technique required for my radiation, and whispered my own silent prayer that He make each 13 second count go smoothly. 13 seconds. It isn't long at all. Yet on the radiation table, it feels like eternity. In the comfort of my own home, with my stopwatch to challenge me, I can hold my breath for a full thirty-three seconds... without really even trying. As a young kid in the swimming pool, I could hold my breath even longer. So, anxiety is the only explanation...that and the mouthpiece, nose clip, and machinery rotating above me. Yes, fear is what makes these few minutes of treatment so difficult. Fear of another mass is what made this weekend so difficult. And, again I am reminded of the quote that I chose to uplift me at the start of this cancer journey. *"Let your faith be bigger than your fear."*

The wisdom of this story: Take a deep breath and let it go.

One Week After

Thursday, March 24

One week after my first chemo, when I boasted that chemo wasn't really too bad; my blood pressure took a dip which caused me to fall, which required me to get an x-ray of a very tender arm. The arm was fine, but we all know how the story goes from there, chemo *(still haven't found a nice way to say it)* kicked me in the ass. One week after my first radiation, when I boasted that radiation wasn't really too bad; I did something to hurt my hip/back/thigh. Delighted that my post-chemo hair is fighting hard to grow, I felt it necessary to shave the tiny bit of stubble that had appeared on my legs. My already not-so-good-hip *(hip dysplasia at birth)* hadn't been kicked up onto the shower bench for a shave in several weeks. It was a stretch to get it up there, but I didn't think I was doing any harm. I felt an uncomfortable twinge later while getting dressed, but was still okay. I taught all morning, even had lunch duty, and did fine at my radiation appointment. I felt tired when I got home, but excruciating pain in my back/hip/thigh prevented me from sitting down. I think my morning routine, combined with swinging my legs up onto the radiation table had just been too much. When I couldn't even get comfortable in bed, I thought a trip to the orthopedic might be appropriate. I had x-rays six years ago, and I prayed that I hadn't done any recent damage. When you are a normal patient you go for an x-ray, get the all clear, and go home. When you are a cancer patient, some medical personnel tend to flip out a bit. The physicians' assistant *(that's who you see at the walk-in injury clinic)* told me things didn't look quite right with the ball of my hip *(I had only indicated that there were problems with the socket)*. They lost my x-rays from six years ago, so there was no way to make a comparison. The words that followed included recommendation for complete bloodwork, a CAT scan, no let's make that an MRI, maybe it's a fracture, and he wanted everything STAT. I didn't feel the need for STAT, as I was pretty sure this was related to my morning shave. It was at that point when he didn't seem to know what he wanted, I asked for a second opinion *(which appeared to upset him)*. He consulted with a doctor who recommended a full body bone scan. I asked if this was because of something suspicious on the x-ray, or simply because I am a cancer patient. As I suspected, it was only because I am a cancer patient and they wanted to rule out bone cancer, *(and most likely protect themselves)*. I had spent my afternoon crying in both frustration and pain. On a scale of 1-10, my pain was a 10, *and I never admit to that much pain*. The fear of bone cancer terrified me, but I found comfort in knowing I had just completed intense chemotherapy and my oncologist had never suggested additional scans. *And I really was pretty sure this all started with shaving my legs*. At that moment, I learned to stand up for myself and told him there would be no scans until I consulted with my oncologist to see that she deemed them medically necessary. I left with pain meds and steroids, and in a polite way told the scheduling lady that the PA was an asshole who needed a lesson in bedside manner. I called the oncology office in the morning, and was told that full body bone scans aren't typically recommended without symptom or suspicion, but a hip MRI would be appropriate. While I was on the phone with them, the PA called me. Somehow, my missing 2010 x-rays had been magically found. He did a comparison, and only the expected degenerative changes were noted. My pain was most likely a musculoskeletal issue and a muscle relaxer was prescribed. There was no need for bloodwork or any additional scans. In the world of education I compare this to losing student data, assuming the worst, setting forth panic, and requesting unnecessary testing. It would be a teacher fail. While I know that everyone makes mistakes, this was orthopedic fail. I now have copies of all of my x-rays and I will never go back there. I won't let my mind wander to bone cancer, and I will allow only my oncologist determine what scans I need post-treatment. It seems like my confidence about treatment grows after the first week, and then a fall or an injury humbles me. I feel tired, old, and sore. I feel victim to cancer. I'm back to days of pain meds and pajamas...*and it sucks*. I am hopeful this muscle issue subsides so that I can focus on getting through radiation. I told my sweet technicians that I don't care if they have to roll me up on the table—I will not allow my pain to cause me to miss a treatment. Today will be day 7 then 26 treatments to go. My paper chain is getting smaller. I'm closer to being cured.

The wisdom in this story: Don't shave your legs, and learn to be your own advocate.

McFlurry

Thursday, March 24

There is a lot about the radiation treatment that is unpleasant...the awful gown, a sore body being shifted on a hard table, and the timing of gated breathing. There is the machinery that moves around you, the button to press, and the aloneness you feel when the technician leaves the room. However, in comparison to chemo, it is not awful. Some say that obese people reward themselves with food. I never really wanted to believe that until today. I have had seven radiation treatments and seven McFlurry ice cream treats in as many days. It helps take the taste of the plastic breathing tube out of my mouth. I know a stick of sugar-free gum would do the same, but I like the sweet reward of the McFlurry best. Most people I know are thinking that swimsuit weather is just around the corner. Even if I could get this body swimsuit ready, my tender skin won't be ready for the sun. And so I will indulge. There are 803 calories in an Oreo McFlurry, but I'm not counting calories, I'm counting radiation days. In the end, I will have enjoyed every bite of 33 McFlurry treats. I won't begin to admit to how many jelly donuts...

The wisdom in this story: Sweet treats make even the worst days better.

Dry Your Tears

Wednesday, March 30

My father never wanted to see his daughters cry. Even a single tear streaming down a cheek was met with the words "Dry your tears." It wasn't a gentle, reassuring "Dry your tears," but rather a direct order that such nonsense needed to stop. However, my mother was the one who pulled out the tissues and told us that everything was going to be okay...even when she herself wasn't sure of her words. While I could never understand my father's comment *(and it made me cry even more)*, I understand it a little better now that I am a mom. There is nothing more heartbreaking than to see your child sad. While I'm not quite sure if this was the reason for my dad's seemingly lack of compassion, it does allow me now to forgive him a bit. It is true that much of what we learn as children, we carry into adulthood. To me, it's hard to allow the tears to flow. I bottle up emotion and when I can't take it anymore the floodgates open. I've often thought in my own mind that tears are a sign of weakness. In my forever fight to be strong, I thought I shouldn't cry. I will yell, scream, and curse before I will allow myself to cry. And yet, cancer got the best of me this year....I have cried, and cried, and cried. Some people say that tears are cleansing, but to be honest, I feel worse after I cry. However, even through tears, I have found the strength to keep going, keep fighting, keep on keeping on. Today was radiation treatment number 11 of 33...radiation treatments one third of the way completed. As I look back at the lengthy list of all I have endured, I wonder how I did it without a huge batch of antidepressants, but I know the answer. Faith, family, friends, *and the occasional jelly donut*. My faith *(when I remind myself)* has been bigger than my fear. I am surrounded by a huge network of loved ones, who just like my mom once did, pull out the tissues and tell me that everything is going to be okay. People tell me that I have been an inspiration. They tell me that they view life differently because of me. They tell me that I am teaching others a resilience and ability to be strong when faced with adversity. While these comments are great for my ego, my strength does not come from within. I am wrapped in your love, and through tears, I thank each and every one of you for being there for me through these most difficult days. You have held on tight, and refused to let go, even when it may have felt like I was pushing you away. 22 more treatments to go and I'll be planning a jelly donut party. We have a lot to celebrate, and I will probably cry. What should you bring, you ask — tissues.

The wisdom in this story: People cry, not because they are weak. It's because they have been strong for too long. (unknown)

Non-Stop

Thursday, March 31

Today was a good day. I received some great radiation news. It has been a rough week with my hip/back/thigh pain, but I was determined to let nothing get in the way of my daily radiation treatments. My technicians have been incredibly patient, helpful, and kind as I position my poor pathetic self on the table each day. It is evident that they are experienced in working with the elderly, crippled, and frail.

So, today was Doctor Day. Once a week, I am examined by the doctor. We review my treatment plan and discuss concerns:

Fatigue: not awful *(I'm pretty proud of that, so I left out the little detail about my two-hour nap on Tuesday).*

Skin: I have yet to notice a significant difference *(slathering on the stinky-smelling lotion several times a day must be working).*

As with everything else throughout this process, I have no idea what to expect. *(Well, I do suspect tenderness, redness, itchiness, and even blistering could occur — but have no timeline to guide me.)* So when the doctor asked if I had any questions, I asked, "So, my skin. Is it looking as you would expect at this point in my treatment?" He smiled, and answered, "Much, much better." The nurse echoed his words. Now, this could mean one of two things. It could mean that by this time next week I will be miserable, or it could mean that the stinky-smelling lotion is protecting me nicely and I will continue my radiation non-stop through May without difficulty. I'm praying for the latter. One day at a time. Each day I feel a little less defeated and closer to being cured.

The wisdom in this story: I can do this...

See You Tomorrow

Tuesday, April 5

It takes a special person to be a health care professional. I spend my days surrounded by special people. There is an incredible amount of math and science, physics to be exact that goes into a radiation plan. The doctor oversees it all; the nurses care for my physical and emotional well being; and the technicians are responsible for precisely placing my body on the table so that tattoos and lasers are aligned perfectly. *Every single day.* I still vividly remember the first day of my radiation treatment. I was terrified. I fought hard not to cry as I lie motionless on the table. With hands cradled behind my head, I was unable to move, let alone wipe a single tear. I focused intently on proper breathing and matched each breath to the counts the technician spoke into his microphone. And then it was over. As I left the room, the technician's cheerful voice followed with, *"I'll see you tomorrow."* Ugh. Tomorrow. While I knew radiation treatments were going to be daily, it wasn't until that exact moment the reality of going there every single day hit me. I went back the next day, and was greeted by the office staff, the nurses, the doctor, and the technicians... *again.* I have done this every day since, 16 times to be exact. Tomorrow will be number 17, past the halfway point of 33 total. While I still dislike going, and I sometimes still have to fight hard not to cry *(every step of fighting cancer is emotional)*, I have grown to love the people who care for me each day at one o'clock. I tell the technician I'm not fond of hearing him say, *"I'll see you tomorrow,"* and he simply laughs. Deep down, I know that each and every day brings me one step closer to being able to use the word cured. One step closer to never having to walk through those doors again. I am so ready to bring this chapter to a close...

The wisdom in this story: The health care professionals I am privileged to know have given me the promise of a whole lot more tomorrows.

Broken Crayons

Sunday, April 10

Sometimes I think I was a little odd as a child. Probably a little OCD before such a diagnosis was ever made…but only OCD about some things. While my bedroom was a disaster, *yes I mean a disaster*, my crayon box was more manageable. My box of school crayons was perfect. My tiny hands held my crayons delicately and I colored in long even strokes. While other kids' crayons became lost or broken, I was proud of my neatly kept set. I always put my crayons back into the box in the order of my favorite colors:

> *purple*
> *blue*
> *red*
> *green*
> *yellow*
> *orange*
> *brown*
> *black*

I memorized and could say that list in order quickly, reciting the colors effortlessly. Kindergarten plus 12 years of school, four years of college, a Masters degree, and 26 years of teaching….*I am what they call a lifelong learner.* For as long as I can remember, I have put my perfect little crayons in their perfect little order, in my perfect little box. In the top drawer of my teacher desk, I still keep my neatly organized eight. However as I grew up, I realized that very few children care for their crayons in such a way, hence the reason I describe myself as a little odd. I vividly remember teaching my oldest child how to color. He had his own framed "gallery" on my kitchen wall when he was just two. He was a rough and tumble boy. It was far more enjoyable for him to put crayons in his tractor wagon than to actually color with them. While my hands were always tiny and delicate, his toddler hands were chubby and huge. We called them bear paws. He held those crayons tightly, and they quickly became broken. His bright blue eyes looked for my reaction, and I calmly told him that broken crayons still color. I had learned this early in my teaching career. Even though broken crayons still color, it pains me a little to see them *"not so perfect."* My life this year, fits nicely with this story. I met recently with another cancer patient. I adore her. Her story is similar to mine, and she is a great source of comfort to me. We talk a lot about how our lives have changed since diagnosis, and most certainly not in a good way. She suffers from long-term side effects from both chemotherapy and radiation, and me — well, I'm just still trying to figure out how I feel. I'm no longer the same sick I was with chemo, and my complaints thus far about radiation are fairly minimal, but I still don't feel like myself. In one of our conversations, we talked about feeling tired, old, and broken. I feel very emotionally tired, somewhat physically tired. My body lacks the energy to give me what I call the youthful *"swing in my step,"* so I feel old. Lately, it's hard not to notice the brokenness. As I faithfully apply the radiation cream to my breast and underarm, I am reminded of my large lumpectomy and lymph node scars. Just today, I noticed a more visible skin darkening which is a sign of reaction to radiation. While I'm proud that my hair is starting to grow, I'm still "bald enough" to feel the need to cover it. I haven't worn mascara since the '80s, along with some bright blue eye shadow, and my once beautiful lush eyelashes are thin and often tear-filled. Not the sad tears, but the chemo-tears that seemingly never end. I'd be lying if I said the sad tears don't come — there are plenty of those, too. While it sounds vain to be complaining about my physical appearance when I will soon have good health, it is sad and frustrating to me. I am comforted in knowing that most women would probably feel a little broken, too — if they had walked the path I have this year. People tell me they love my happiness, my attitude, my strength. I think of my crayon colors, and how even at a young age I favored the more cheerful colors in a box of eight. Even in my vast assortment of crayons at home, I favored the pretty ones: periwinkle, sky blue, carnation pink, and the most beautiful silver. I liked brick red and cadet blue, which I thought were strong colors. But, who in the world would actually choose to color with burnt orange, or worse yet raw sienna and burnt sienna? Then there were orange-red and red-orange, colors that just confused me. When I think of life with cancer, it's a little like my disastrous childhood bedroom, something over which I didn't seem to have control. Before cancer, I lived my life much like I organized my perfect little crayons — in a perfect little order, in my perfect little box. For a long time, it was all sky blue and such. I found strength in the richer colors as I needed to, but cancer — it was pure ugly and confusing. Things are not so perfect, but life isn't supposed to be perfect. It pains me a little to see the brokenness. In time, I will pick up the pieces and this year will just be one distant memory, sort of a blue gray, or maybe sepia. Everything will be okay.

The wisdom in this story: Broken crayons still color.

Terra Cotta Pet

Monday, April 11

There is nothing I find more annoying than the terra cotta pet commercials. *Well, maybe the noise of the machine during an MRI is more annoying.* Not maybe, definitely. But, the terra cotta pet song is a close second. Terra cotta pets became popular when I was a child, and as much as I remember about my childhood, I can't remember ever having one. To be honest, I can't remember ever wanting one. But my son wanted one several years ago. He didn't want one, he *begged* for one. I bought one, but told him they were a joke. The instructions state that sprouts are to grow within a couple of weeks to resemble the animal's fur or hair. *His never sprouted.* We had a bald terra-cotta creature in our home for months until the whole entire thing magically disappeared. My last chemotherapy treatment was on February 11. The oncologist told me the chemo drugs would be out of my system in about three weeks. I don't think I completely agree, as I still have teary eyes, some slow to heal chemo-sores, and somewhat limited taste buds. I still suffer from chemo-brain *(either that or I have become very forgetful since my February birthday)*. However, around the middle of March, my hair slowly started to grow. I was thrilled! I called the first sprouts white or light gray, my hairstylist called them blonde, *(bless her heart)*. No, I wasn't there for a hairstyle, I was at the salon for a hug. When you go to the same salon for years, the stylists become family. About a week later, some dark stubble appeared. *(I think my kids prayed about this so I couldn't continue to blame them for the gray)*. With every little hair that emerged, I breathed a sigh of relief. Current lawsuits exist for one of my chemo drugs. Apparently, some patients who receive it suffer permanent hair loss. In December 2015, the same month as my first chemo infusion, the FDA amended its safety labeling of the drug to note that *"cases of permanent alopecia have been reported"* after usage. So yes, my hair is growing, and I am thankful. A permanent hair loss would simply always be a reminder of my cancer...*awful, awful cancer*. As my hair grew, I was determined to do all that I could to speed along the process. I visited a beauty supply store and purchased a shampoo/ conditioner/treatment set specifically designed to promote hair growth. As I rubbed my scalp with the products in the shower, the terra cotta pet song popped into my head. Was this shampoo a joke? A fifty-dollar joke? Time would tell. Two weeks have passed, and while I still look mostly bald, the amount of hair is promising. I do believe the hair products are working. Maybe by summer I will look like I have a very short buzz cut. For now, I am happy with what little hair I do have. My principal made it very clear that she always wants me to feel comfortable at school. I mentioned no longer wanting to wear a hat. She was wonderfully supportive. So today, as my students gathered at the door to enter the classroom — I approached them. I was greeted with the most enthusiastic and happy voices from the children. They are so busy learning about growing things in science, that the language one student used to describe my hair made me laugh out loud. He exclaimed, "Mrs. B is growing hair!" Not Mrs. B's hair is growing, but Mrs. B is growing hair. Again, I thought of the terra cotta pet. I had NO hair, so my hair wasn't growing, I was growing hair. Children are very loving, caring, compassionate, and resilient, and if anything they are happy with my "new look." We talked about how my treatments will end the last day of April, and we started planning a huge pink party for May. It felt delightful and refreshing to no longer have a sweaty and itchy hat covered scalp. In my classroom today, I felt my smile brighten and my eyes sparkle.

The wisdom in this story: I am blessed to work at a wonderful school, with an incredible staff and adorable students.

Haircut by Choice

Wednesday, April 13

I took my daughter to the gym tonight, and while there another mom came in and stood beside me. She had a very short haircut in the back *(which she later said was a clipper blade two)*, and it was only slightly longer on top. She was very attractive, and the first thought that popped into my head was *very short haircut=cancer survivor*. She smiled pleasantly and I found myself looking away. She enthusiastically said, "I don't know if your haircut is by choice, but I wanted to tell you that it's very flattering. I would love to have that hairstyle." Now, I need to remind you that my scalp is still very much visible, and it's not even close to a style any woman would want. So, I could only assume she was either a cancer patient like me, or was for some reason curious about my condition. I told her that the haircut was not by choice, and mentioned my diagnosis and treatments. She said that her short hair *was* by choice, that she just liked it that way and didn't have time to be bothered doing her hair. And then she went on to say that she lost both her father and aunt to cancer, and has another aunt newly diagnosed with breast cancer. While I could have been offended that this complete stranger wanted to ask me such personal questions, the conversation flowed freely and I enjoyed her company. It turns out that our daughters are in both the Wednesday and Thursday classes together. As the girls have gotten older, most parents drop off, so I don't really know any moms. Chatting with her was nice, and reminded me of times at the gym when my girls were in elementary school. When we parted ways, I told her that my hair would probably be longer, and hers would probably be shorter the next time our paths crossed. We both giggled. Since December, I've noticed the hair of women everywhere. I've thought about colors, styles, and the bangs I miss so much. I have admired practically everyone I see, and long to have something to brush again. When you are a cancer patient, you feel right at home in doctors' offices where everyone looks tired, worn, and bald just like you. To go out in public takes courage. While people never intend to stare, they do, and sensitive people like me easily become self-conscious. So whether the *"your hairstyle is flattering"* was genuine, or simply a way to learn more about me — I'm appreciative of the way the stranger at the gym reached out to me. It was so much better than a stare.

The wisdom in this story: Someday again soon my hairstyle will be my choice. I'm seriously considering a clipper blade two and only slightly longer on top.

Spring Cleaning

Saturday, April 16

My husband loves Fall. My mother always loved Spring. I love the change of seasons, but I was never able to choose a favorite. I love Spring-cleaning though. While my full energy for cleaning hasn't returned, I had some important things on my list for today. Since December, a large basket on a corner table in my bedroom has held hats...warm winter hats, cancer-ribbon embroidered ball caps, athletic beanie caps, bandeaus, and knit hats handmade with love. While I am glad that my hair is growing, and happy with my decision to no longer wear hats, sorting them was a little emotional. I made a pile to donate to a thrift store that specializes in items for cancer patients, but some I will keep forever. There is the fleece sleeping-cap that my oncology office encouraged me to take, to protect my tender scalp as my hair fell out. There is the hot pink bandeau that I bought with every good intention of embracing the color that represents breast cancer — *I never wore it.* There is the *"Love Your Melon"* hat that was a gift from a special family on a day that I most needed a friend. There is a set of three knit hats from the department store that I favored until the weather became warmer. There is the pastel pink knit cap that was lovingly made by my coworker's mother. I wore it for my driver's license picture and everyone told me I looked cute. I will have to look at that "cute" picture for the next three years. *Damn you licensing center for not allowing chemo patients to use previously taken license pictures.* At least the hat was nice! There is the online-ordered white hat made with too much fabric that made me look like a chef. There is the black hat made of incredibly soft bamboo material. While I loved the comfort of that hat, I hated the look. From the front, I looked like a bad-ass-biker-mama; from the back the rosettes made me look like a 95-year-old woman. And then, there is the first hat I received as a gift after diagnosis, from a friend I met years ago. People tell me the color compliments my eyes, and the embroidered "*Life is Good*" logo makes me smile. As I carefully placed these special hats in a beautiful, decorative box, the morning sun shone brightly through my windows. My daughter placed the box high on my closet shelf where I keep other special things. I stepped outside on this bright warm day and looked at a backyard full of yellow dandelions. I love spring and the new life it represents...weeds and all. I will treasure the months of summer perhaps more than ever before. They tell me I should be free from chemo side effects six months after my last treatment—just in time for Fall. I will slip my hand into my husband's hand and suggest we go for a Fall walk. I will have plenty of hats from which to choose as the weather becomes cool and crisp…and I will tell my husband that I like Fall best. Life is good.

The wisdom in this story: To every thing there is a season, and a time to every purpose under the heaven: A time to weep, and a time to laugh; a time to mourn, and a time to dance. Ecclesiastes 3:1, 3:4

Not Quite Sun-Kissed

Monday, April 18

As a young child of the '70s I spent most of my summer days outdoors. I bypassed sun-kissed quickly, and my mother laughed at my golden brown tan. I never really got a sunburn. I was just brown. I remember a summer vacation at the beach when the rest of my family complained about sunburn. I remember being curious about what if felt like to have a sunburn. They all groaned and called me lucky. As I got older and spent less time outdoors, I experienced sunburn. *Ouch.* As a young twenty-something I fell asleep in the sun, and got a sunburn that ended up blistering. I was miserable. So when I heard people compare radiation to a sunburn, I said: "*I'll be fine with a burn, I'll be fine if it's itchy, I'll be fine if it peels....I just hope it doesn't blister.*" As things haven't always gone my way with this cancer journey...my skin has blistered. In fact, I'm not really sure you would call it blistering. I bypassed pink, red, golden brown, and tan...I went straight to black. I bypassed itchy, peeling, and blistering...I went straight to raw. However, in the grand scheme of fighting cancer, it's not awful. Black and raw skin is still better than chemo. Even though my skin is tender to the point it is uncomfortable, I'm not miserable. The area of reaction is still minimal. I'm one of the fortunate ones. I'm still functioning — still going to work, still doing happy things in my role as mom. The radiation nurse gave me a medicated gel-pack to wear. It should help with the healing. It will be awhile before my skin is ready for the summer sun.

The wisdom in this story: The raw will heal, the black will fade, and someday I'll stay outside just long enough to get a light sun-kissed look that makes my smile shine more brightly.

A Little Donut

Wednesday, April 21

I don't know when my affinity for donuts began, but I have many fond donut memories. Call it a comfort food, call it an addiction, donuts are always there. When I was a child, we would travel about four hours to visit my grandmother. Less than an hour into the ride, my father would ask if anyone wanted to stop and "get a little donut." *(My mother always laughed at this, because it was her preference to drive straight through, and how could anyone possibly need to stop after less than an hour on the road).* As a 16-year-old, I remember being trusted to drive the car down the road from my grandmother's house to the donut shop on the corner. I delighted in being the first awake and out the door to "surprise" everyone with donuts. My grandmother loved jelly donuts, so I suppose that's why I loved jelly donuts. In college, I did something that I'm almost embarrassed to tell. I carpooled with another student teacher to our placement about 20 miles away. We met at the donut shop. Lunch at our school was family style, and fish sandwiches were often on the menu. We both *hated* fish sandwiches. On fish sandwich days, my carpool friend and I treated ourselves to a dozen donuts. We chose apple and spice and told ourselves they were *healthy.* We ate donuts the whole way to school. Then we stopped on the way home at a great little milkshake shop for a large chocolate milkshake. While donuts remained a part of my life, *and I secretly delight in having a husband who sneaks out on Saturday mornings while all are still asleep and brings home donuts,* my real donut "addiction" didn't start until my cancer diagnosis. It was early in my story, a day when I planned to go to church, but ate a jelly donut and spent the remainder of the morning in bed feeling sorry for myself. Friends who read my story empathized, and I have since received more than a dozen donut shop gift cards from sweet friends. In December, a donut shop opened in the small town where I work. Now, I must preface this with the comment that this small town has many banks, pizza shops, and car dealerships. A donut shop was a BIG deal. *(Maybe not as big of a deal as the Wine and Spirits shop that opened earlier last year, but nevertheless, a big deal!)* The location wasn't ideal, the parking lot maze a bit complicated, and I doubted I'd ever go there…but now I think I'm considered a *"regular."* It started with smoothies when that was all I could tolerate during chemo. Then one day, I added a donut to my order. I didn't think I could handle my favorite jelly donut, so I opted for chocolate frosted. It was heavenly. Sometimes I buy a box of six and share with a dear friend and coworker at school. *Okay, she eats one and somehow the box becomes empty by the end of the day.* We talk about things not related to cancer or school, and wipe the chocolate from our faces before the students arrive. For now, donuts are one of the only things that taste really good. While I know that my donut addiction is a dietary nightmare, I am not currently dieting, I am a cancer patient. I have enjoyed every bite of every donut. As cancer treatments end, and my taste for healthier foods returns, I will choose juicy fruits over jelly donuts. I will choose fresh greens over frosted chocolate. I will remember the dieter's philosophy of everything in moderation and eat one donut instead of five — but during treatment, donuts were always there. Maybe they were a comfort food, maybe an addiction. Someday, my frequent donut shop visits will simply be another fond donut memory…but not before I host a donut party, and you are all invited! Details will be announced soon!

The wisdom in this story: There are 270 calories in a jelly donut. Ditto for chocolate frosted. Sigh.

One Day More

Thursday, April 22

I love Broadway. My daughters love Broadway. We are a farm family, but we also love the adventure of the big city — New York City. Taylor Swift sings, *"Welcome to New York, it's been waiting for you."* Then there's the old familiar, *"Start spreading the news, I'm leaving today,"* written by Fred Ebb. My anticipated end-of-radiation date was Friday, April 29...a total of 33 treatments. I am scheduled to accompany my daughters on their high school choir trip to NYC the next day. I couldn't think of a more perfect way to celebrate the end of my treatments. Today was Doctor Day. The doctor told me I had seven treatments to go. *I corrected him...no six.* Surely there must be some mistake. *I have been counting. Carefully. Every single day.* No, seven. It seems that the doctor can choose either six or seven boost treatments. For me he has chosen seven... **34** treatments total. While I dread having to go for an additional treatment, I am glad that my doctor is treating the tumor area aggressively. So, instead of finishing next Friday, I will finish the following Monday. I will still go to New York. I will enjoy every minute. But I will return home to one day more of treatment. It reminds me of one of my favorite songs from *Les Miserables.*

"One day more.
Another day another destiny.
This never ending road to Calvary.
These men who seem to know my crime,
will surely come a second time.
One day more."
(Herbert Kretzmer, et al)

I will sing my own words:

One day more.
Another day another destiny.
This never ending road to cancer-free.
Bad cells who know how hard I fight,
will never come a second time.
One day more.

The wisdom in this story (from my other favorite Les Mis
song, one word changed):

"Do you hear the people sing?
Singing the song of angry men?
It is the music of the people
Who will not be <u>sick</u> again!

When the beating of your heart
Echoes the beating of the drums
There is a life about to start
When tomorrow comes.

Will you join in our crusade?
Who will be strong and stand with me?
Beyond the barricade
Is there a world you long to see?

Then join in the fight that will give you
The right to be free."
(Herbert Kretzer, et al)

You just sang that...didn't you?

You Are Invited

Sunday, April 24

Two-hundred-one days ago I received the news of my cancer diagnosis. From that day forward, the word cancer became a bit all-consuming. For 201 days I have been fighting cancer, both physically and emotionally. While I continued to live my life as wife, mother, sister, teacher, and friend there have been bumps in the road. While I once boasted about my independence, I relied heavily on my husband to tend to my wounds, aches, and every need. While I was once the mom who lovingly cared for my children and never missed any of their events, my children lovingly cared for me while I had to pick and choose which events I felt well enough to attend. My sister. *Well, let's just say I don't know how people get through life without a sister.* My worries were her worries, her wisdom my strength. One day at a time, with my sister there for me always. While I was once the teacher that could make the struggling student laugh at his mistakes and learn without even realizing it; I became the teacher who had to quickly dry my tears before the students entered the classroom. They learned in spite of my illness, substitute after substitute guiding their path; and never failed to greet me with warm smiles, hugs, and shouts of "Mrs. B is back!" when I returned after lengthy absences. A friend once gave me a CD of her favorite songs to listen to during my treatments. One of the songs was *You've Got a Friend in Me, (Randy Newman for Disney's Toy Story)*. That song made me laugh and cry all at once. The catchy tune mixed with deep emotion was a great song for someone fighting cancer. Rachel Platten's song *Stand By You*, brings tears to my eyes every single time I hear it. Cancer is ugly. I was never quite myself during this journey, and I will never quite be myself again. I discovered a favorite quote during my illness, "*If you want to find out who is a true friend, screw up or go through a challenging time and see who sticks around,*"(*Karen Salmansohn*). I am blessed to have so many wonderful people who have never left my side as this awful disease called cancer became all consuming in my life. I am blessed to know that so many wonderful people have read my stories and walked this journey with me, holding my hand, praying, and offering words of encouragement. I have six more radiation treatments to go. While my future will be filled with appointments, examinations, tests, and scans, the hardest part of my fight is almost over. I am ready to celebrate, and all of you are invited to join me at my house for a jelly donut.

Please mark your calendar!

Date: Monday, May 16

Time: 7PM.

Details and more information about how to RSVP will follow soon.

The wisdom in this story: (from Rachel Platten)
"Oh, tears make kaleidoscopes in your eyes
And hurt, I know you're hurting, but so am I
And, love, if your wings are broken
Borrow mine 'til yours can open, too
'Cause I'm gonna stand by you."

Something Missing

Monday, April 25

I like order. I like structure. I like routine — almost to a fault. *Okay, most definitely to a fault.* I find comfort in routine, and I don't always embrace change. The first 27 of my radiation treatments were almost exactly the same. I entered the waiting room, wrote Michele B on the clipboard, and took a seat, *my seat*, beside the tropical fish tank. A technician came for me, and escorted me to the changing room where I learned to quickly remove everything waist up and sloppily tie the blue gown. *I learned that changing quickly means less time there altogether.* I tossed my clothes in the locker, presented my patient ID card to be swiped, and entered the room. Each time the technicians worked ever so gently and carefully to ensure that my body was properly aligned on the table for treatment. Once aligned, they left the room and I focused on my breathing. The ladies counted like this:

Push your button.
This is your first normal breath.
This is your second normal breath.
Take a breath and hold it.
13-10-7-4
You can breathe.

This repeated two more times *(always starting with 13 but often ending with fewer counts.)* Then the big machine rotated and there were three more sets of countdowns. The male technician counted differently. His counts were 13-11-9-7-5, now you may breathe. While one might think I would prefer his counting backwards by two, for some reason his way made the 13 seconds seem longer. But the teacher in me liked his use of *may* breathe as opposed to *can* breathe, so I guess that made up for it. After the final countdown I would hear the technician turn off the microphone. A squeak of the door would follow, and I would be finished. While I love all three of my technicians, there are specific things I appreciate about each of them. One lady has an unbelievably calming presence and a beautiful smile. Her reassuring nature helps with my anxiety. The other lady sometimes whistles, and just seems genuinely happy. It's hard not to smile when she is around. The man has a habit of saying "Here we go!" as he exits the room to begin my treatment. I wonder if he even realizes he says it, *and I also wonder if he secretly pretends he is an amusement park ride operator offering me a pleasant send-off.* The last seven boost treatments specifically target the tumor area, so my routine as I knew it has changed. While the careful positioning on the table remains the same, I am no longer required to breathe through the snorkel-like breathing tube. No more button, no more counting, no more microphone— just me, alone, on the table wondering how soon it will be over. I'm learning to listen to the noise of the machines, trying to learn the timing of the new routine. *Thank goodness the door still squeaks.* I felt a little out of sorts today. While I know it's because I haven't learned the new routine, there was something more…something missing…and then I realized. Two of my waiting room friends finished their treatments last week. One elderly gentleman was my favorite. He smiled with his eyes and always told me he was praying for me. He was fighting a fight much harder than mine, and was brought in a wheelchair by various members of his loving family. His daughter once told me he said I was "such an encouragement to him," but I think it was the other way around. I truly looked forward to seeing him each day. His daughter took our picture together on his last treatment day. I wish I had thought to ask for a copy. I missed my friend today. The waiting room was quiet…*too quiet.* I miss the comfort of my old routine.

The wisdom in this story: In the world of cancer and shared experiences, strangers quickly become friends.

The Pink Notebook

Thursday, April 28

Today is Doctor Day and my mind is flooded with questions. I will meet with my medical oncologist this morning, and my radiation oncologist this afternoon. Once again, the pink notebook has emerged from my cancer basket and I will write a list of everything I want to know. I will print neatly, and methodically check things off as the doctors answer as much as they are able to answer. No one will really have all of the answers, especially to my biggest question, *"Am I really cured?"* However, I found much comfort in scheduling my breast surgeon appointment for the end of May. The receptionist called it a Survivorship Appointment. *Survivorship. Survivor.* What a blessing to know that those words are now a part of my medical vocabulary. Life is good!

The wisdom in this story: "Let your faith be bigger than your fear." (unknown)

The First Year

Friday, April 29

Yesterday was a good day. My medical oncologist told me that no additional scans *(other than mammograms of course),* are medically necessary. I will take a pill for the next five years, but risk of cancer recurrence is low. I asked her if I was allowed to use the word *cured.* While I loved her honesty, I hated her answer. She showed me a curve based on research that outlines the chance of recurrence. She calmly explained that while chance of recurrence is low, there is never a *zero* percent chance. She said that cured isn't really a medical term, and doctors prefer to use the word remission. And then she smiled brightly and said "But, *survivor.* You can use the word survivor. You are most definitely a *survivor.*" I asked if I had to wait for my mammogram result to have my port removed, and she eagerly said, "No, let's get that out..." and just that simply, I was given permission to get rid of the very last reminder of some of my sickest, saddest days. I will schedule the procedure as soon as possible. My hair continues to grow and my radiation wounds are beginning to heal. On the outside I'm beginning to resemble my pre-cancer self. However, on the inside I'm still tender, emotions are still raw. While I cried a few tears in the doctor's office today, I didn't openly address my emotional struggles. But, she knew. *Good doctors just know.* I didn't have to tell her that cancer still felt all-consuming in my life...she already knew that, too. She told me that the first year is the hardest, as is with any life change. She said that for awhile, I will question every little ache, pain and body difference. She said my mind will immediately wonder if anything that seems out of the ordinary is cancer. Then, in time, it will become easier. She said someday I will forget about it. Now, while I doubt I will ever forget about it, I do believe that it will become easier. Once again, I reflect back on my sister's words. One day at a time. Piece by piece, step by step, my life will fall back into place again. I will feel whole. This journey with cancer will always be a part of me. Others told me life would change for the better as a result of having gone through this experience. I can't say that is true. I still feel like I have spent an entire school year fighting cancer. I feel like I lost a whole school year. But someone recently said, "but look how many years you have gained..."

The wisdom in this story: "You have to fight through some bad days to get the best days of your life." (unknown)

New York

Saturday, April 30

Welcome to New York, it's been waiting for ME!

The wisdom in this story: The sun will come out tomorrow.

Eight Streets and One Avenue

Saturday, April 30

Considering I've spent most of the past six months in various stages of rest *(chair, couch, bed)*, I'm proud to say that it felt good to walk eight streets and one avenue in sunny NYC. I'm back. Almost.

The wisdom in this story: "Turn your face to the sun and the shadows will fall behind you." (Maori Proverb)

Hakuna Matata

Saturday, April 30

Intermission at *The Lion King* and my eyes seem to be floodgates for tears. Music has always evoked great emotion for me, but being on a trip I wasn't sure I would be able to take; seeing the one Broadway show that has always been on my bucket list; and listening carefully to the lyrics...I realize that there is so much to be learned from a Disney show:

Hakuna Matata!
What a wonderful phrase.
Hakuna Matata!
Ain't no passing craze.
It means no worries
for the rest of your days.
It's our problem-free philosophy.
Hakuna Matata!
(Tim Rice)

The wisdom in this story: Those two words will solve all of your problems.

Bright Lights, Big City

Saturday, April 30

Cruising down the Hudson admiring everything about the city I love, I can't help but be reminded of the airplane pilot who safely made an emergency landing on the Hudson in 2009. Just as his hands so carefully and precisely guided his aircraft in such a way that lives were spared, my doctors have carefully and precisely managed my care. Because of their expertise, I am able to enjoy this evening with too many teenagers on the dance floor, very loud music, and the best dinner cruise I've taken in years. They will remember this trip forever, and thankfully I will, too. Chesley Sullenberger III, the pilot on that flight, has since written a memoir. He is the author of a New York Times best seller. The book title is today's wisdom and sounds like a great summer read.

The wisdom in this story: "Highest Duty: My Search for What Really Matters" (Chesley Sullenberger).

Rain

Sunday, May 1

It has rained all day, but our time in NYC has been filled with shopping on 5th Avenue, singing, and dancing. Life is good!

The wisdom in this story: "Life isn't about waiting for the storm to pass, it's about learning to dance in the rain." (Vivian Greene)

Shades of Pink

Monday, May 2

I awoke to the most beautiful, lavish, and fragrant floral bouquet from my husband, pink vase and all. While I love the flowers, the heartfelt note from him meant even more. I am blessed. While he says that I am a remarkable woman, I truly couldn't have gone through all of this without his love and support.

The wisdom in this story: "When someone has to fight cancer, the whole family and everyone who loves them does, too." (Terri Clark)

Got Tissues?

Monday, May 2

Donut Party
My Home
Monday, May 16
7:00 PM
All are invited!
Please wear: pink
Please bring: tissues

Today was my last day of treatment. I am ready to celebrate:

-two-hundred-nine days of fighting cancer

-mammogram

-breast ultrasound

-breast biopsy

-hearing a nurse say *"yes, it is cancer."*

-hearing a doctor say *"but it is curable."*

-diagnosis of Intermediate Grade Invasive Ductal Carcinoma

-genetic test, BRCA1/2

-breast MRI

-sentinel node injection

-lumpectomy surgery

-sentinel lymph node biopsy

-re-excision surgery

-bottles of pills

-Oncotype DX test

-recurrence score report of Highly Aggressive cancer

-hearing a doctor say *"you need chemo."*

-medi-port procedure

-countless bags of chemo drugs

-three injections

-one on-body-injector

-cherry Italian ice and strawberry smoothies

-fluids for hydration

-one bag of potassium

-hearing a radiation oncologist say, *"Forget about chemo. Chemo is over."*

-twenty-seven traditional radiation treatments

-seven boost radiation treatments

-far too much bloodwork

-four pairs of ugly socks

-fifty-one ugly hospital gowns

-seven tubes of radiation lotion

-thirty-five derma gel pads for healing

-too many tissues

-more donuts than I will ever admit.

While so many praise me for being strong and courageous, I have complained every step of the way, and sometimes about the dumbest things. I hated the socks. The ugly gowns stole every ounce of my modesty, and I never quite knew how to tie them. Worse yet, were the tissues. As I sat in the imaging centers, my surgeon's office, hospital rooms, my medical oncologist's office, and my radiation oncologist's office—I promised myself I wouldn't cry...and in all of those places I cried. And cried. And cried. And then I got mad. I asked my husband why those kind of places have crappy tissues. Women sit day after day filled with worry about biopsy results, or sit in offices hearing news they never want to hear. They endure discomforts, pain, and sickness too difficult to explain to non-cancer patients. While they probably don't admit it, most women cry. And there is nothing worse when you're feeling awful, than a crappy tissue.

One in eight women will be diagnosed with an invasive breast cancer in her lifetime. She will hear the news and dry her tears with crappy tissues. She will try hard to remember a childhood filled with soft brand tissues, as the budget-brand irritates her already swollen eyes. And she will cry more. While many will cry for over 200 days, I am one of the fortunate ones. Most will cry more.

Soon some of you will attend my jelly donut party. Everyone always asks what they can bring. Please bring one box of soft tissues for every breast cancer patient you have known. Maybe I'm the only one you know, perhaps you know several. I will deliver these tissues to the places where I have cried.

The wisdom in this story: Together, we can soften the sadness of those newly diagnosed or those fighting the fight.

Regrets Only

Monday, May 2

I have always loved parties. I can vividly recall helping my mother fill out the invitation cards for my childhood birthday parties. Sometimes we wrote *RSVP* but sometimes we wrote *Regrets Only*. Regrets Only was my favorite. Regrets Only held such promise. Those words meant that everyone you hoped would attend would actually be there, unless they made that dreaded phone call to say that regretfully, they couldn't come. I haven't seen the use of Regrets Only in years. I'm not sure why. Perhaps it became politically incorrect when everything in life had to be politically correct. Perhaps it was inconsiderate and rude to assume that busy people with busy lives had time for you. Perhaps it was respectful to make saying no seem okay. As you know, I'm planning a party. If I say so myself, I can host a pretty terrific party, *(some people think wine and beer is the answer, but nope...its sugar... sweet sugary jelly inside a donut laden with white granulated sugar).* Sugar-filled people are happy people, and my sad story needs a happy ending. My very own dairy princess daughter will be serving rich and creamy whole milk. There will be door prizes and party favors. I have some very special people to recognize and well, it isn't really a party without a party favor. There will be chocolate, too — because chocolate makes everything better. A lot of people read my stories. Only a select few comment regularly. Some say they don't know what to write. This time it's quite simple. In the comment section below, please simply RSVP to let me know whether or not you are able to attend. I would love to say Regrets Only, but I can't take the risk of running out of donuts, or worse yet the risk of too many leftover donuts! While I know you are busy people with busy lives I hope you have time for me. Someone asked if spouses are welcome. Yes. Kids? Yes. As my mother always said, "The more the merrier." Just indicate in your comment how many from your family will attend.

The wisdom in this story: This is my time to give back. My time to thank you for your prayers, your love, and your support.

A Full Day

Wednesday, May 4

It's 1AM and I can't sleep. My mind is spinning as I think about my ungraded writing assessments, the pile of summer copy work that came back early and needs to be filed, and the lesson plans I still need to complete. I had forgotten what it is like to teach for one full...*day*. Then I remember the pink streamers lovingly hung in my classroom doorway; a whole school of students and staff wearing pink *(except of course me, as no one gave me the memo)*; the gift of a beautiful pink floral scarf from my thoughtful principal *(who secretly kept me from getting the memo)*; the faculty room full of pink and the surprise of delicious pink cupcakes to celebrate the end of my treatments; and the hugs, smiles, and "We're so happy for you" comments that filled my day. Then there is the boy—the tiny one who sometimes struggles. He is the one who stuck his tongue out at the substitute teacher because, "She just isn't kind like you, Mrs. B." He lost a tooth. Losing a tooth in first grade is a big deal. His toothless smile helped to remind me how much I love teaching. Tomorrow I will score the writing assessments, file the copy work, and add some brightly colored stickers to my neatly printed lesson plans. I will add more to my to-do list, and feel overwhelmed as most teachers do during this time of school year. But I will see pink, and be reminded that I am so very blessed. Every day is a gift.

The wisdom in this story: Hugs from co-workers, pink cupcakes, and smiles from toothless six-year-olds can fill a day nicely. Sometimes, the lesson planning has to wait until tomorrow.

Pills, Pills, Pills

Thursday, May 5

It is fairly common knowledge that with every drug on the market, there will always be side effects. So when my oncologist suggested that I would need to take a highly controversial drug every day for the next five years, I questioned her. "What if I don't?" I asked smugly. Her answer was simple, "bone, brain, liver, lung." I was momentarily speechless. She followed with, "those are the places the cancer could most likely appear." Speechless again — and for those of you who know me well, that doesn't happen often...okay, ever. *I am never ever speechless.* Even though I was finished questioning, as the thought of cancer anywhere else terrified me, the doctor continued to explain. She told me that some women take this particular drug to ease the symptoms of menopause. Then she asked, "If women take this to prevent menopause symptoms, why wouldn't you take it to prevent cancer cells from growing?!?" *At that exact moment, I decided that yes, indeed, I would be taking that pill — every single day — for five years.* Thankfully, it wouldn't begin until after treatment. I had forgotten about the pill until my follow up last week. At my visit, the doctor took time to clarify even further how the pill will work to block estrogen from attaching to cancer cells. Without estrogen, the cancer cells will disintegrate...simply die. Sounds like a plan! It wasn't even a matter of yes or no, but a direct question from the doctor, "Which pharmacy?" I use a mail-order prescription company for daily medications. I haven't used it in awhile. I felt certain that my credit card on file had probably expired. I wasn't really in a hurry to update my payment information. Just yesterday, I called to provide a new card number. A pre-recorded message told me that my prescription had already shipped. *So much for my efforts to procrastinate.* The bottle of pills arrived today. I took a deep breath, said a quick prayer for no side effects, and swallowed the first of what will be 1,825 pills total. It's going to be a long five years.

The wisdom in this story: The only way to beat cancer is to accept the reality, embrace the pain, and find the courage to move forward, one day at a time...

Labels

Saturday, May 7

My best friend's son has autism. About the same time we were becoming friends, I learned professionally that it is best not to call a child autistic, but rather to refer to him as *a child with autism.* The teacher who shared this with me is an expert in her field, and stressed the importance of putting the child before the disability. I often think that is why I was able to connect with my friend and be a support to her on difficult days. I always saw her son as a child first. When she called to tell me about some of the crazy things he did, I often told her "that's not autism—that's just boy." I knew because my son *(who does not have autism)* did some of the same crazy things. When I was first diagnosed with breast cancer, I hated hearing the words "you have cancer." I was easily identifiable as a sick person with my swollen face, tired eyes, and lack of hair; but when people unknowingly asked about my condition, I struggled to say "I have cancer." I found it much easier to say "I am a cancer patient." But in saying that, I was putting the cancer first. While I openly admit that cancer became all-consuming in my life, I was still me. I was still the loving, kind, caring, and compassionate person people know and love. I often worried that when people looked at me they saw only the cancer. My oncologist assures me we did everything medically necessary to clear my body of the cancer—I am now cancer-free. I absolutely adore my friend's son. He is a great young man—*with autism.* Autism isn't who he is, he is a great young man first. I read once that cancer patients often identify themselves with their greatest pain, because it is also their greatest victory, but I refuse to let my cancer identify me. I am not my cancer. I am not a cancer patient. I do not have cancer. It is past tense...I *had* cancer. I *was* a cancer patient.

The wisdom in this story: Believe it or not underneath the

pain, the sickness, and the sadness, I was always just me.
Thank you for loving me always.

Mother's Day

Sunday, May 8

My mom was absolutely the best mother. She died almost 15 years ago, and not a day goes by that I don't miss her terribly. She was the one who was always there. She delighted in being mom and grandma, and her life was far too short. My children have missed out on being loved by her. Her smile was contagious, and she was what I call *"gushy."* She never stopped telling us we were wonderful, but she wasn't afraid to delicately point out our flaws either. She loved hugs, kisses, and together times. She was happiest when a child or grandchild was by her side. We talked for hours. While I always miss her, Mother's Day is especially difficult. While I'm blessed and proud to be a mom, I miss *having* a mom. It is a very bittersweet day for me. On Mother's Day, so many like to ask how one will celebrate. *Will there be breakfast in bed? Will there be flowers? Jewelry? Cards? Will you go out to dinner?* While all of these things are nice, and the television commercials never seem to stop telling us so, to me Mother's Day is really just about *being the best mother.* It is about being the one who is always there. It is about being delighted to be a mom. It is about smiling and being gushy. It is about telling my children they are wonderful, while delicately pointing out their flaws. It is about hugs, kisses, and together times. It is about having a child by my side and talking for hours. Because of my illness, it was hard for me to do some of those things this year, but I think my kids understand.

The wisdom in this story: Today I will celebrate the lady who taught me how to be a mom, and the children who called her Grandma.

The Photograph

Monday, May 9

My mother always refused to have her picture taken. After her diagnosis, she allowed it a bit more, but she still didn't like it. Sadly, I have very few photographs of my mother. At some point in my life, and I can't recall when, I started to refuse to have my picture taken. I can't speak for my mother, but in speaking for myself, I think it's all about self-image. When people struggle with obesity, no matter how happy they are on the inside, they aren't usually happy with how they look on the outside. If they avoid photographs, and mirrors, they are allowed to feel flawless and just let their inner happy shine. I have a whole lot of inner happy. As my oldest daughter gets ready to graduate from high school, I have spent countless hours sorting through old photos for her graduation scrapbook. Occasionally I come across one of myself, smiling with my husband or gazing lovingly at a child. I like what I see. I don't see the baby belly that never went away *(and I know it's really a jelly donut belly)*. I don't see the once slender young woman who now carries around way too much extra weight. I don't see the bad hair day, or the mismatched mommy outfit. I see happy. I see the happiness that I have always felt inside. As I sort through the photographs, I quietly comment and seek affirmation from my husband, "*gosh, I look young; look how skinny I was in this one; I loved this hairstyle; look how happy I looked.*" I found a family picture taken at my daughter's princess pageant just five days before my diagnosis. My thick hair was blowing in the wind and my lips were parted widely as my smile was really more of a laugh. *I looked happy. I was happy.* My daughter recently had her Senior Prom. We hosted pre-prom pictures at our house. After the usual father-daughter photo, my husband took the camera and suggested we needed a mother-daughter photo, too. I complied. The girls posed happily for photos, their dates willing, but slightly uneasy. In the days of selfies, I don't think it was the photographs the boys disliked, but the whole idea of prom in general. When it was almost time for the kids to leave, some of the moms became a little tearful. This was just one more high school milestone for our babies. Someone suggested a photo of all of the moms. *I cringed.* But I have just survived the year from hell and managed to come out with my inner happy intact. *For the scrapbook. I would agree to a photo for the scrapbook.* Then, one mother posted it to a social media site. I was thrilled she didn't tag me. When I looked at the picture, I wondered why I hadn't dressed more appropriately for the weather. I wore capri pants and sandals, the other moms wore long pants, sweaters, and sensible shoes. I was almost the shortest in the group, and most definitely the heaviest. In an effort to be comfortable and to appear slimmer I wear my clothes baggy. In the photograph they look sloppy. Even on a damp rainy day, all of the other moms had beautiful hair. I had...*none*. Well, okay...maybe enough to cover my bald scalp. My head was tilted slightly and somewhat awkwardly, as if I didn't know which camera to look toward. I think in my mind I was secretly avoiding the camera altogether. *For the scrapbook.* In a day or so, the social media world will have forgotten about the photograph, and it will find a spot amongst many others in my daughter's prom scrapbook. Yesterday, my Mother's Day was wonderful, and early in the day I thought it would be nice to have my photo taken with my kids. But my older two were both working, and it was late in the day when I remembered. By then, I had already removed my bra, *(one of the perks of recovering from radiation is the doctor's orders to go bra-less as often as possible).* My early-morning lipstick had faded, and I was wearing my old, poorly fitting eyeglasses. *Nope. No picture. Maybe next year.* Yes. I will look better next year. It was just before bedtime when my oldest daughter slid a beautiful gift bag across the table toward me. She said, "I wanted to give you this at dinner, but I forgot." I opened the bag and tried hard not to cry. She had framed the mother-daughter prom day photo of the two of us. She looks like a younger version of me. She looked stunning in her Cinderella blue gown and bright eyes sparkling. Her hair and makeup were just perfect. Her smile just happy. Incredibly happy. I looked more closely at my image in the photograph. I didn't notice the clothes too spring-like for the rainy weather. I didn't notice that I was the shortest and the heaviest. I didn't notice that my clothes looked baggy, sloppy. I didn't notice my lack of hair or somewhat awkward head tilt. I noticed *happy*. My inner happy was shining. I was just happy. Incredibly happy. The framed photograph will be placed in a special spot on my dresser. I will treasure it always.

The wisdom in this story: The best part of being a cancer survivor is being there for every one of your child's milestone moments. While the memory will never fade, it is always best to take a picture.

Last Visit

Monday, May 9

Today was port-removal day, a day which in my mind officially signaled the end of the nightmare I have lived since the 24th of September. Of course there will be mammograms too many to count, five years of pills, and occasional sleepless nights in my future...but those pale in comparison to what I have endured throughout the last several months. As on previous hospital visits, my sweet husband dropped me off at the door and then left to park the car. I was greeted by an overly enthusiastic but adorable twenty-something hospital employee whose personality reminded me of my son. He informed me he would escort me to Outpatient Registration. The hospital is under construction and my usual path to the elevator had been rerouted. I thought it was odd that he even rode the elevator with me, but I suppose they can't take the risk of someone like me daring to brighten up the place with a can of spray paint concealed in a purse. I told the young man I thought his job would be an interesting one, escorting patients who arrive grumpy and depart groggy. He laughed a sweet, respectful laugh, and was probably calling me crazy lady under his breath. As I thanked him for helping me find my way, I mentally added him to the list of individuals who in one way or another have been part of my path to cancer-free. At the registration desk I had the same receptionist I've had for each of my outpatient procedures. She scanned the same cards, I signed the same consent forms, and I waited in the same waiting room. The noise of contractors working held promise that the hospital I love to hate may someday have a brighter future. I was greeted by a familiar nurse and taken to a familiar room. On the bed was an oversize hospital gown and a bright yellow pair of socks. I changed quickly and relied on my husband to help me with the ugly socks. I tend to get

228

cold in the hospital, so I suggested he put them over top of my own pink ribbon breast cancer socks that I hope to never wear again. There was the IV nurse I didn't particularly like. When I told her that the IV team usually said I was a tricky patient she said, "I'm sorry to tell you that you're not all that unique like a unicorn, most people have tricky veins." *What the hell? A unicorn? No, I didn't like this nurse.* After a painful stick that proved to be an unsuccessful attempt, she admitted defeat, politely excused herself, and brought in an expert IV team nurse. I suppose she went off to dream of unicorns, because I never saw her again. It took a bit of effort, but the IV team nurse found a good vein on her first attempt and I reminded her that she was the best. Another nurse came and attempted to draw blood. She looked slightly distraught until my IV angel appeared again and offered to assist. A couple of vials of blood later I was transported down the hallway for the procedure. As usual, the tears started before I even met the doctor. I told the sweet nurses that one might think medical anxiety would have subsided a bit after all I have endured, but I'm still a mess. They assured me everything would be okay, and they would make sure I was plenty sleepy. I remember feeling more of the cut than a sleepy person should feel, but after that the procedure went as planned and seemingly to me without incident. I later learned that my heart rate was again a problem, but only for about ten minutes and my blood pressure remained stable. They kept me for vitals checks longer than I would have liked. They gave me a pain pill that reminded me how much I dislike pain pills, and they gave me a wheelchair ride to the car. I thought the moment would feel monumental, like the closing of a door. It didn't. So many thoughts were running through my mind as we drove away. Mostly, I was thinking that while I'm sure the newly renovated hospital will be nice, I'm not in any hurry to go back.

The wisdom in this story: Thoreau once said, "Go confidently in the direction of your dreams. Live the life you've imagined." I'm ready to live.

Time to Make the Donuts

Thursday, May 12

Dunkin' Donuts' sleep deprived Fred the Baker was featured in television commercials for 15 years. Those commercials always made me laugh. The phrase, "Time to make the donuts" became one my mother would sometimes say when I was up and out the door early in the morning.

Tomorrow morning, bright and early, I will place our Monday donut order. I am hopeful that you can come to celebrate with me.

I watched one of the vintage Fred the Baker commercials online. It shows him repeatedly coming and going.

"It's time to make the donuts.
I made the donuts.
It's time to make the donuts.
I made the donuts."

I felt a little like Fred the Baker during radiation.

It's time to go for treatment.
I went for treatment.
It's time to go for treatment.
I went for treatment.

But just as the radiation doctor taught me to say, *"Don't say chemo. Chemo is over,"* I have learned on my own to say, *"Don't say treatment. Treatment is over."* It is time to celebrate!

The wisdom in this story: My sister always told me to take things one day at a time. I discovered that one jelly donut at a time was even a little sweeter.

Rainbows and Butterflies

Friday, May 13

I needed my windshield wipers for my drive to work this morning, and it remained dreary most of the day. Recess was held indoors, at a time of year when children really need to be outside. Today was Sidewalk Chalk Day for my class. Teachers say that we plan these special events during the last few weeks for the children, but selfishly we look forward to the fun days just as much. I spent most of the afternoon stealing glances out the window in hopes of dry sidewalks before bus time. Shortly after three, the sun was shining brightly and students enthusiastically lined up at the door carrying baggies of sidewalk chalk. Some children had none, and others had enough chalk to draw for miles. We assembled quickly, each student sharing a sidewalk square with another. The only instructions given were to have fun, share chalk, and stay in your space. Students drew fervently, as they knew our outdoor time was limited. They drew rainbows, hearts, butterflies and images of the sun with yellow and orange rays. They wrote their names, played tic-tac-toe, and laughed out loud. In spite of the hues of pastel all around me, my eyes were drawn to a dark puddle on the blacktop. The water rippled gently in the breeze, and I wondered why this bit of water had not cleared. It appeared that a parked car had blocked the warm winds and bright sunshine. And of course, I thought of cancer. Some of my days were like puddles of darkness, cancer blocking the warmth and sunshine we so desperately need. Those days were made bright only due to the gift of God's love and the prayers of many. My port incision is tender, more so than I would have expected. But on the sunny side of things, my oncologist seems confident that I am cancer-free. As my students lined up to enter the building, I admired everyone's artwork. In spite of the rainy start to the day, the sun prevailed and we enjoyed our Sidewalk Chalk Day. The projected rain in tomorrow's forecast will wash it all away, but there will always be plenty more chalk to share.

The wisdom in this story: Sometimes on the dreariest of days we need to make our own rainbows and butterflies.

A New Beginning

Monday, May 16

Today will be a day of celebration. I'm hosting a pink party for my students and their families. Each student will receive a *Tough Kids Wear Pink: I wear pink for Mrs. B* t-shirt. There will be four bags of balloons to toss around the classroom. There will be pink refreshments, and a time to simply laugh and be silly, something our tight curriculum doesn't always allow. We will revisit the cancer lesson I shared with my students so many months ago, and we will agree that while there are awful things about cancer, there are also good things, great things. While I'm still trying to convince myself that there are really good and great things, I can be a VERY persuasive teacher and the kids will walk away from all of this with a happy perspective. Tonight I will relax and be myself with the people who know that cancer has been my awful, and managed to love me throughout this journey. We will eat jelly donuts and chocolate frosted donuts. We will eat cherry Italian ice — the only food I could tolerate during chemo, and what kept me hydrated, something so very crucial during treatment. We will take silly pictures, write scrapbook memories, and celebrate survivors. There are ten breast cancer survivors in my circle of friends, and sadly one who passed away that I will always remember. I will laugh, I will cry, and I will thank God for blessing me with so many good people in my life. Then, the party will be over. This is my last story. I will wake up tomorrow and each day after feeling thankful to have come out on the other side of all of this still smiling. As the mother of a princess, and sometimes affectionately called queen, I find this quote especially fitting:

"One day she finally grasped that unexpected things were always going to happen in life. And with that she realized the only control she had was how she chose to handle them. So she made the decision

to survive using courage, humor and grace. She was the queen of her own life and the choice was hers." (Queenisms)

I have done my best to live this year with courage, humor, and grace. But sometimes I fall — and I have learned:

> *The first to help you up are the ones*
> *who know how it feels to fall down.*

Thank you for reading my stories. Thank you for loving me no matter what. I'm going off to live my happily ever after, and appreciate knowing that you will be by my side.

The wisdom in this story: When I look in the mirror I see scars, both physical and emotional. But I realize after all those hurts, scars, and bruises, after all of those trials, I really made it through. I did it. "Scars simply mean you were stronger than whatever tried to hurt you." (unknown)

The end.
(but really, there's more...)

Me Again

Monday, May 16

This morning I wrote that it would be my last story. I guess I needed just a little more closure. So here I go again. The donut party, *if judging by the donuts*, was a success. I purchased 12 dozen donuts. There are exactly ten donuts left. Not ten dozen, ten donuts. Now, many of those were taken in to-go boxes and I did see a gathering of some teenagers/young adults at the donut table for an extended period of time, but to say that 134 of the 144 donuts are gone from my house is a good thing. I am deeply humbled by the presence of so many who came to celebrate with me. I will forever be appreciative. While I felt compelled to talk a bit, I hope it wasn't too long. While I wanted to recognize each and every one of you personally, it meant a lot to recognize the cancer survivors. How wonderful to close in prayer, as it is truly the prayers of all of you that helped to sustain me. *And then the tissues – so many tissues.* I thought it was a cool idea...give someone fighting the fight a softer tissue to dry the tears. What I didn't realize, was how deeply emotional the tower of tissues was for so many of us. I watched as some of you wrote the names of loved ones on the labels, and I saw the tears in your eyes. Cancer truly does affect everyone. One friend's eyes welled up with tears when she walked into the room. We collected 231 boxes total, and my school faculty and staff have pledged $50 toward the purchase of more. I will begin making deliveries tomorrow. And then there is the *what next*. Two of my friends have invited me to join their breast cancer awareness fundraising teams. I didn't want to hurt their feelings, but I'm not quite ready. I was proud of myself that I was able to be honest and say so. I can talk to people for hours in the comfort of my own home, but to walk a lap and call myself a Survivor, sounds a little overwhelming to me. I pour my heart out in my stories, yet I like to remain a little anonymous. I'm more of a behind the scenes kind of girl. Maybe I will offer to help with fundraising. This time next year — for $25 a person, you can enjoy a jelly donut and what one friend called the biggest chocolate frosted donut she has ever seen. You can enjoy the company of some really good people. We can build an even bigger tower of tissues, and pray together for a cure. Maybe, just maybe, there will be a book signing.

The wisdom of this story: I can't wait to see what comes next, and next, and next.

The Happily Ever After

Friday, May 21

There seriously might need to be a part two of this book, as writing has become such a part of my life. I woke up today with enough hair to call it *"bed head"* or almost enough to call it a *"bad hair day."*

The wisdom in this story: Treasure the bad hair days. It's God's way of reminding you that you have hair.

The Rose Bush

Wednesday, May 25

My mother had the most beautiful pastel pink miniature rose bush. In my first few years of teaching, she clipped roses for me and put them in a tiny crystal vase. "For your teacher desk," she said with a smile. My mother didn't quite understand that crystal vases and a classroom full of six-year-olds wasn't necessarily the best mix, and she insisted they would look pretty at school. I took them to school. I loved those roses. The vase survived. A few years after my mother passed away, my father made plans to remarry, and put the house up for sale. *It wasn't just any house – it was my childhood home.* To some people who have a more transient lifestyle, a childhood home isn't really a big deal. But I spent more than 20 years living in that house, and every nook and corner *(both indoors and out)* held a memory. Selling my childhood home was a big deal. So one sunny day, my husband and I, shovel in hand went to the house and told my dad that we wanted to dig up the rose bush. *Too late. He told us we were too late.* It seems that the realtor had already taken photographs of the house and property, and it had to be sold exactly as it had been advertised. *Really? According to whom? A potential buyer would notice the absence of a rose bush?* I thought he couldn't possibly be serious…but he was serious. He was being difficult. Under my breath I called him a selfish asshole. Okay, maybe I said it loud enough for my husband to hear. I cried. My dad and I argued. He won. I like to win. I was bitter for years. At one point, I was even tempted to knock at the door and ask the new homeowners if I could buy the rosebush from them. The new homeowners didn't tend to the flowerbeds in the same way my father had. Things looked overgrown and full of weeds. Unkempt. I drove past the house often, and I cried. The tears weren't really about the rosebush, the tears were about the connection to my childhood that now seemed missing. When my husband and I built our new home, I carefully described the rosebush to our landscaper — *tiny pastel pink blooms on a miniature bush.* He told me he knew exactly what I wanted. I was surprised and a bit disappointed when I came home to see a whole row of bright pink rose bushes. They were small, but not the miniature and not the color I had wanted. *I wanted to say tear them out, I wanted to say it wasn't okay...but again, I knew it wasn't really about the rosebushes.* These were okay, even pretty — just not what I wanted. I have hated those rose bushes for eight years. Just last year, I told my husband I thought I wanted to tear them out. Today is my follow-up appointment with my surgeon, and they called it a Survivorship Appointment, which thrills me. They said to allow about an hour for the appointment. I'm not quite sure what could possibly take an hour. I pulled out my pink notebook, the pink notebook in which I have carefully documented each and every appointment. My notebook is the color of my mother's roses. Most notebook entries include questions. So I started to think about my questions — long-term questions one might want to ask a doctor responsible for the surgeries that removed the cancerous tumor from my body. While I still consider myself a little emotionally fragile, I am almost completely physically healed. My scars, while prominent, are beginning to fade. There are of course lumps, bumps, and things I never noticed before that don't feel quite right, and never will. My oncologist already explained my long-term prescription. She already explained the protocol for mammograms and scans post-treatment. So questions for the surgeon...I wasn't really sure I had any to ask. I walked outside and sat down with my notebook. The pink rosebushes distracted me from my deep thoughts. *They were beautiful.* Some small buds, some roses in full bloom, each delicately blowing in the gentle breeze. They are the bright pink color I've loved to hate this cancer year. It was only then I realized that perhaps I truly am at peace with all of this. Perhaps I truly do feel like a survivor. Perhaps my mind that was once overwhelmed and spinning with questions too numerous to ask, has found the calm after the storm. Perhaps even though the rose bushes weren't what I really wanted, I have learned to find the beauty in them after all. My daughter has three days of high school left before her graduation. She will go to college, and in four short years she will be an elementary teacher, hopefully with a classroom of her own. She will need roses for her desk. They will be bright pink, and I have the perfect crystal vase in which to put them. If she ever tells her daddy she wants to dig up the rose bush, the answer will most definitely be "of course."

The wisdom in this story: Seek to find the beauty in everything, even if it's not exactly what you wanted.

Survivor

Monday, May 30

I struggle with the word *Survivor*, and I really didn't understand why until today. I am reluctant to use the beautiful survivor gifts I have been given *(mug, keychain, necklace, magnet for the car, etc)*. I'm not quite ready to walk the Survivor Lap at our local event. When someone calls me a survivor, I feel myself blush a little. Just today, I realized why. While the words Cancer Survivor have beautiful meaning *(cancer gone from the body, end of treatment, a healthy prognosis)*, in life everyone is a survivor in one sense of the word or another. I think of childbirth. The pain was intense, but the gift of new life so very precious. I survived childbirth. I think of young children learning to walk. They stumble and fall, only to get up again…and again…and again. They survive. They take off running. I think of my youngest daughter who just earned a fantastic score on her Geometry final exam. Both her brother and sister struggled in Geometry, and she felt certain she would fail. Not only did she survive a challenging class, a less-than-favorite teacher, and a difficult final exam, she came out shining. While I take pride in my incredible kids, and know that my husband and I have raised them well, I think of my sister. She raised her three children on her own, as a single mom. They are wonderful young adults and I can proudly say that my sister survived the challenges of motherhood that simply exhaust most of us — and she did it smiling. On this Memorial Day, I think of other mothers, who see their children grow up and choose to serve our country. On a daily basis, those mothers must survive the thought that their children may never come home again. I think of those serving. Survivors. Each and every one of those young men and women who do return home have survived the unimaginable. I once read a quote that states, *"Be kind. For*

everyone you meet is fighting a battle you know nothing about."
(Ian Maclaren) I think of this quote often. We are all struggling
in our own way, and in the end we all find ways to survive
what challenges us. Cancer challenged me. With the help of an
incredible team of medical professionals and the prayers of
many, I survived. Yet, Survivor isn't a word I am comfortable
using. It's not that I don't recognize that I fought the fight. It's
not that I don't feel incredibly proud. It's not that I don't find
myself sometimes repeating the words, *"I did it!"* It's just that I
like to try to be a little humble. As my children were growing
up, I always told them they could brag and boast at home, and
it was my job to appreciate that they were truly fabulous. But
outside of the home, I gave them a simple reminder...*keep your
pride inside.*

**The wisdom in this story: I am a survivor, but it is okay if I
choose not to openly call myself one.**

Growing Up Together

Tuesday, June 7

Thirty years ago today, I met my husband. He had sparkling eyes, a great smile, and hair that he liked to "spike," which was quite popular in the '80s. If I say so myself, I was a skinny little eighteen-year-old with a fabulous wardrobe, beautiful hair, a great deal of confidence and the whole world ahead of me. We were both quiet in our own way, and loud when silly *(and angry)*. My wit and his charm seemed to be a comfortable combination. We built a pretty incredible life together with careers we love, a warm and friendly home, three fantastic kids, and more pets than I care to count. Our lives were guided by faith and we tried *(not always successfully)* to bring out the best in each other. People tend to say that we grew old together, but I prefer to say that we grew *up* together. Throughout the years, my husband became nearly bald. It bothered him more than it bothered me. I gained a lot of weight and started to wear frumpy clothes. It bothered me more than it bothered him. Together we shared life's disappointments and sorrows, but my husband never lost the sparkle in his eyes or his sweet smile. Even when life knocked me down, I maintained the confidence needed to endure. But somehow, through it all, my laughter became a little lighter, my soul a little sadder. *And that was before the cancer.* Life wasn't always easy. I blamed my seriousness on growing up. We watched other marriages dissolve and saw our loved ones die. We watched people we never thought would leave our lives walk away and never look back. We saw jobs that were easy in our twenties become challenging in our forties. We saw bills too many to pay, and responsibilities too many to bear. We tried to make all the right decisions as parents, and wanted to raise our children to become better versions of ourselves. We were simply exhausted just trying to face the challenges of each day. *And then came the cancer.* My husband's sparkling eyes looked scared. His sweet smile softened. The surgeries, chemotherapy, and radiation treatments wreaked havoc on my body. I lost my hair and it bothered both of us. My once-vibrant self faded and I became *the sick person.* And then, almost as quickly as it started, the cancer year ended. Life started to return to normal, even though none of us really knew what the new normal would look like. People told me that cancer would change my life. I didn't want to believe them. However, I now admit that in a very small way, I am beginning to view life a little bit differently. I am realizing that I still have the whole world ahead of me. I am realizing that while it's okay to sometimes be quiet, loud when silly is much better than loud when angry. I am realizing that I have a pretty incredible life. I am looking forward to spending a relaxing summer with the man I fell in love with so many years ago. We have some amazing teenagers in our lives who love to laugh out loud. They are the perfect combination of wit and charm. And while my husband no longer has hair to spike—I do—*and it's almost the length for a perfect Mohawk.*

The wisdom in this story: Don't let the challenges of life lighten your laughter or sadden your soul.

Here I Am

Monday, June 13

All three of my children have perfect smiles, a gift from a very
talented orthodontist. It pains me when they don't regularly
wear their retainers, and it pains them when they wait too
long between nights of wear. I was a kid who never had any
orthodontics past the initial consult. For those who may recall
that I am a medical wimp, that fact of never needing braces
was a good thing--*a very good thing*. My sister wore the awful
headgear *(do they even DO that anymore?)* followed by braces,
rubberbands, and a retainer *(I think)*. The fact that I don't
clearly recall whether or not she ever had a retainer probably
means that she didn't wear hers faithfully either. *(And even
though she seems to recall far less than I do about our childhood
days, she will probably tell me she wore her retainer)*. Anyway, just
because I didn't need braces, doesn't mean that I had the
perfect smile. I had a space between my two front teeth. "It's
simply cosmetic," the orthodontist had said. "It can be fixed,
but only if it bothers her." At the age of needing braces, I don't
suppose it ever bothered me, but I do know it made me feel a
little self-conscious. Maybe I didn't always smile the widest
smile, but I was happy in so many other ways that the smile
didn't matter so much. However, the older I got, the gap
seemed to bother me a bit more. I knew adults who were
getting braces. I would *never* get braces. *Medical wimp.* Yep. I
did cancer. But braces, no way. And a retainer...never! I have a
niece who has a gap between her two front teeth. When she
was braces-age, she was told the same thing I was told years
earlier. But this kid has spunk! Her answer was much better
than mine. She told her mother that she was afraid she
wouldn't like her *new* look after braces. The gap between her
two front teeth defined who she is, and without it, she just
wouldn't look like herself. That is one of the things I have

always loved about this special niece. She has a confidence that surpasses that of most adults *(at least that's my opinion of her)* and she has always marched to her own drummer. As a young child, she chose sneakers over sandals and they were *boy* sneakers to be exact. It never phased her that her boy cousin sported the same pair. She chose tie-dye over summer sundresses and didn't attempt to impress anyone. She has a "here I am" attitude and her commitment to family warms my heart. She faithfully checked in with me during my illness, and wore her heart on her sleeve. Her brother encouraged me in my writing and her sister brightened my days with her giggles. It was hard for them to see me sick. *It was hard for me to see me sick.* Cancer changed me in so many ways—simply cosmetic, things that can be fixed, but only if they bother me. I look in the mirror and I see scars. While the scars themselves don't bother me, the reminder of cancer does. My once bald head now has what some people call a very short impressive-looking haircut. To me, it is yet another reminder of cancer. It's growing out, all in its own time and all in its own direction. My once smooth skin now wrinkles in places I didn't know I had wrinkles. My forehead wrinkles in a disapproving scowl and makes me look angry when I'm not. My eyes look so very tired. *I am still tired.* Cancer tired. Chemo tired. Radiation tired. *"Sick and tired of being sick and tired"* tired. But then there's my smile. The gap is still there, but it doesn't bother me. I am simply happy… happy to be alive, happy to be finished with treatment, happy to have a really beautiful prognosis, happy to be one of the fortunate ones.

The wisdom in this story: All of these things put together, the scars, the hair, the wrinkles, the tired eyes, and the smile define who I am now. I have a confidence that surpasses who I was before and I no longer attempt to impress anyone.

Busy Doing Nothing

Monday, June 20

I thought I was doing great. I finished work exactly one week ago today. The very next day was my daughter's college orientation. That evening, my out-of-state cousins came to visit for a few days. While they were here, one cousin observed me in the kitchen and commented that I cooked a lot. I answered, "I like to cook." Truthfully, I have simply learned that I like to be *busy*. Any kind of busy—busy doing anything. Busy doing nothing. When I am busy, I don't *think*. When I do think, I think about cancer. Today was the first day in a long time that I haven't been busy. I stayed in bed far too long, and avoided housework and errands. Throughout the morning, I had trouble focusing. By midday, I found myself in tears. I have every reason to be happy. The cancer is as close to being *gone* as possible until confirmed by my September mammogram. Yet, I find that I'm still not feeling quite myself. My joint pain seems worse than I had anticipated. I want to believe it's the weather and not the chemo. My radiation wounds are healed yet still tender. My energy level is a little low, which they tell me is *normal* for up to one year post-treatment. I am mindful of my moods and sometimes feel a little out of sorts. Some say the long-term medications I must take can affect emotion, but I feel *normal enough* not to be overly concerned. My joy today was in making *(or helping my husband make)* a birthday cake for my son. My son is 20. He is an amazing young man. Just the thought of making a cake exhausted me. Now, I must first say that for the past 19 years or so, his cakes have been store-bought and then lovingly decorated by me with cake-toppers like tractors, trucks, and race cars. For some reason today I felt the need to make one from scratch...both cake and frosting. It wasn't the best, which I pray is just the slow return of my taste buds, but he was happy and appreciative. I couldn't be more proud of this special young man I call son. He is a high-energy individual and always has been. When he was a young toddler, I loved to just sit and watch him. He was always on the go. My mother used to laugh at how busy such a little one could be. She called it *"busy doing nothing."* Tomorrow begins yet another calendar-filled week for me. I will be busy, and for that I am thankful. But after this week I will have to learn how to be busy doing nothing. Because I thought I was doing great, but on the not-so-busy-days I'm not so sure.

The wisdom in this story: It is in the quiet moments that the word cancer returns to my thoughts.

Follow Up

Wednesday, June 29

Today is again a doctor day. Oncologist. I will return to the place that knocked me down the most, only to feel thankful that they helped me to be where I am today. It seems that my calendar is quite full of appointments during the next several weeks. In addition to my cancer-related appointments, there are other appointments, too. During my treatments, I canceled dentist, eye doctor, routine physical, and annual gynecology appointments...and now I'm trying to squeeze them into my summer. It's almost overwhelming. A letter arrived in the mail to remind me that it's time for my every-five-year colonoscopy*. I like to think that it's a precautionary measure due to my mom having been a stage 4 colon cancer patient, but I know better. In 2006, they removed a small polyp. Research says that it takes about 10 years for a colon polyp to become cancerous. So yes, as much as I hate the prep, I go for my colonoscopies. It seems that summer gets shorter every year, and this year I have as many appointments as there are weeks. It makes me unhappy. Then I think back to a time not so long ago, when I was lethargic on the couch. It was a time when I didn't eat for days and struggled to stay hydrated. It was a time when I felt like I was just going through the motions, watching my family's life from a distance. It was a time when I hated treatment, but I hated cancer more. It was a time I never thought I'd be able to endure, but my sister's advice of one day at a time made it more tolerable. As I look ahead to my many appointments, I question a bit every doctor's need to follow up, and can fully understand why people choose to delay appointments. But, as I look at my calendar, I am reminded that I would never want to turn the pages back to all that happened this year. So, off I go. I will be the happy, smiling, healthy looking patient in the waiting room. However, I will always look with compassion *(but no sad eyes)* toward the patient who is following their most difficult path. My heart will always ache for the cancer patients and their loved ones, and I will never stop praying for a cure.

The wisdom in this story: No one likes to go to the doctor, but it is something we must do.

*I went for my colonoscopy on August 3rd and the doctor removed a very small polyp. I said a prayer of thanks that routine screenings are available to us. My mom was surely smiling down from Heaven.

In the Moment

Sunday, July 3

I don't talk a lot about the what-ifs, and I don't reflect a lot on all that has happened. I try to live my life in the moment. Yet, sometimes those thoughts come to the forefront of my mind, and I know that no matter how hard I try not to let cancer become all-consuming, it will always be a part of my life. I have always been one who wonders about the pattern of sleep dreams and nightmares. Why do we dream what we dream? Why do things come to us in the night, that we can't always acknowledge during the day? Why do our biggest fears become real in our nightmares? I dream enough to have learned that my dreams are often a mix of things that I think about in real life, but all blended together. While the combination makes my dreams seem crazy, I often wake up just shaking my head. Yet, other times my dreams feel more like nightmares and even at my age I wake up crying. Yesterday, when my husband and I talked about how hard this year has been, I told him if I had a do-over I would have stopped working and focused only on my treatments. I then quickly followed that comment with, "but I pray I never have to do any of it again." I said those words just as I was driving across the river bridge, and looked across the water to see the most beautiful, shades-of-pink sky. Once when my kids were small, my youngest told me that Grandma *(in Heaven)* painted the sky for us. I remember those words with every beautiful sunrise, sunset, and rainbow. I think of tears from Heaven when it rains…and on sunny days, I feel the warmth of my mother's love. I go this week for an annual gynecological exam. *Disclaimer — my stories seem to have moved beyond bras, boobs, and biopsies.* As my cancer was an estrogen positive cancer, we will talk about hormones, menopause, and of course the concern of any gynecological cancers. While I'm not worried, the appointment has been on my mind. Some women who have been diagnosed with breast cancer choose a more aggressive treatment plan and schedule hysterectomies, but I have never been one to choose an elective surgery. So last night's dream that caused me to wake up crying involved these two things: mestasticization and my mom. In my dream, *which is more suitably called a nightmare,* I learned some upsetting news from the doctor. I was told that there was more cancer, and there was a lot. The locations included my other breast and more. The doctors and I discussed my prior choice of lumpectomy vs mastectomy. We discussed the aggressiveness of my cancer. In my dream, everyone around me knew the news except my family. In my dream, I told my mom, who was still very much alive. As her eyes filled with tears, I told her bravely, "I fought it before, and I will fight it again." At that moment, I woke up. I thought of Rachel Platten's *Fight Song,* and started to cry. The dream addressed a fear that is always with me, but one I don't choose to acknowledge during the day. The dream reminded me that I am brave, and as the song goes, "I've still got a lot of fight left in me." I can't live every single day of my life wondering if the cancer will return—but, I can tell myself that if it does come back, I will be ready. For now, I'm just trying hard to live in the moment.

The wisdom in this story: My mother isn't just a sky painter, she is the wind beneath my wings.

The Cheer Bow: A Reprise

Friday, July 8

From the time I was small, my world has been very black and white. There is no gray. I either like you or I don't. If you hurt me, it is hard for me to forgive. While I'm not proud of it, I openly admit that I hold grudges. I forgive, but I never truly forget. This is all perhaps my greatest flaw. I have spent most of my adult life praying to be more accepting, more forgiving, more willing to simply let it go. My youngest daughter is so very much like me in her black and white world. She is spunky and tough, and I've always said that no one will ever shit on her. *(Sorry, there is no nice way to say it).* My older daughter has always been very different. I always said I want to be like her when I grow up. She was always accepting, forgiving, willing to let it go. She was never one to hold onto hurts. She saw the good in everyone...*until this year.* This was the year that she realized not everyone in the world is kind, thoughtful, and caring. *(And this was the year she most needed kind, thoughtful and caring.)* I watched her world become more black and white with very little gray. I watched her hurt because of the actions of others and I saw her struggle to forgive. While she wouldn't admit it, I saw her holding grudges, being angry, and then simply not caring at all. It hurt me...a lot. One of my greatest flaws now passed on to my child who had always been so resilient and lovely. Yet, I knew I couldn't take all of the blame. *Cancer was to blame.* Cancer doesn't just happen to the patient. Cancer happens to the whole family. It was my daughter's senior year of high school, supposed to be the best year, and cancer interfered. She was struggling, and quite frankly, some of her friends just sucked at being friends. In the end, she learned the value of true friendship, but there were a few friends who simply got lost in the shuffle. It was more important for them to fit in than to stand up for her, and that's really okay, because I'm not sure she would be able to stand up for them had the situation been reversed. The less they seemed to be there for her, the less she seemed to care. But I know deep down in her heart, her world isn't my black and white. I know some small part of her wants to find a way to forgive. So I find it necessary to lead by example and pray that she will follow. You may recall one of my deepest hurts, *The Cheer Bow (January 30)*. It was a story about feeling left out and it evoked a lot of emotion from my readers. I heard from many, many people, via posts, messages, even phone calls. But I never heard from the one "Cheer Bow Mom" I called friend. I knew she read my stories, and questioned how she could let time pass without finding it in her heart to acknowledge that I was hurting. It never occurred to me that perhaps she was hurting, too. My written words, my freedom to express myself, were hurtful to her. We were both hurting, but in different ways. In the months that followed, our paths crossed not often, but occasionally. We were cordial, polite, formal, yet underneath it all was the bit of real friendship peeking through. I had always enjoyed her company, and I believe she enjoyed mine. We helped one another pass the time with dinners out while our girls were at cheer practice, and at times shared mother-daughter adventures. *Cancer changed that. Cheer bows changed that.* Things became a little awkward between us, but we never completely lost touch. A text here and there turned into dinner out. We talked, and talked, and talked…and finally, I mentioned the cheer bow story. We laughed a little, but I felt a little sadness and I suspect she did, too. When we parted, my world felt a little less black and white. I think I'm becoming a little more accepting, forgiving, willing to let it go. I told my friend I want a cheer bow for Christmas. She said I'm getting one. My daughter will leave for college soon. I will send this bit of wisdom along in her packed boxes. Maybe, just maybe, she will find it in her heart to reconnect with an old high school friend.

The wisdom in this story — Reprise from February 2: When someone close in your life, deep in your heart is struggling, it takes more than just living your life as usual to be a good friend. It requires you to think about them. A lot. It actually requires you to mean what you say and never stop thinking about them. It requires you to think about how your words, actions, and deeds may make them feel. Every single day. Suffice it to say, you know they would do the same for you.

My Own Advocate

Tuesday, July 12

Last week, I had an annual appointment with my gynecologist. I was dissatisfied with my office visit, and wanted to walk out but convinced myself to stay for the necessary exam. I'm still upset. As my last entry was about "letting things go," I decided that I need to let it go, but not before I write a letter to my doctor's office. This letter was sent today via e-mail to their patient advocate. I've said it before, and I'll say it again—cancer stole my filter. My letter follows:

To Whom It May Concern:

My name is MTB, date of birth XX-XX-XXXX and I have been a patient in your practice for 23+ years. I am writing to share my recent dissatisfaction with an annual visit. First, I must share that my visit was slightly delayed this year due to an October breast cancer diagnosis. I needed surgery, a re-excision, a port procedure, chemotherapy, and radiation. I completed my treatments on May 2. Suffice it to say, I spent most of the past school year *(I am a teacher)* fighting cancer. It was my own personal kind of awful. There was a great deal of physical pain, sickness, and discomfort, and most certainly a lot of emotional struggle as well.

Throughout my many years with your practice, I have seen groups merge, doctors retire, and the name of your practice change more times than I can count. Throughout the years, I have seen doctors' patience wane and bedside manner lack what I would expect as a patient. Near the end of Dr. #1's time with you, he became abrupt, even curt. At that time I switched to Dr. #2, who quite frankly didn't seem to be much better.

Dr. #1 had delivered my first child, Dr. #2 my second child. I admired and respected them both in those early years. I decided that after the year of cancer I had endured, I needed some special care for this year's visit. I selected Dr. #3, who had delivered my third (and youngest) child 15 years ago. I recall that my husband and I were very impressed with him, and in particular the special care that he offered to me as a patient and young mother.

Fast forward to 2016. When Dr. #3 entered his office to meet with me, he asked, "Why are you here?" I thought the question was odd, as my chart should have told him that it was for an annual visit. When I explained that it was for an annual visit albeit slightly delayed due to a recent breast cancer diagnosis, he briefly commented that he had seen a report from my oncologist. I talked with him about the bloodwork *(from my oncologist's report)* that indicated I could be post-menopausal. I talked with him about Dr. #1's previous concern about my irregular menstrual cycle and his recommendation of birth control through menopause. I talked about Dr. #1's concern about pre-cancer cells developing in the uterus due to irregular menstruation. At that point, he stated that blood work showed I was post-menopause, and that there was no concern about the lack of menstruation, nor was there a need for contraception. In wanting to be sure that I understood him correctly, I repeated, "so you have no concern about uterine cancer and feel confident that I am post menopause..." He appeared somewhat annoyed and said, "<u>Yes</u>, I have concern about uterine cancer." He went onto tell me *(in a short and to the point way)* that my obesity and my estrogen receptor pill *(recommended post-treatment by my oncologist)*, put me at great risk for uterine cancer.

Yes, I am obese. The scale clearly tells any doctor that. What the scale doesn't tell is that I already know it. While I don't try to make excuses for my obesity, I don't need it pointed out to me either. The risks — I am already aware that obesity puts me at increased risk for almost everything. I have struggled with obesity most of my adult life. Born with hip dysplasia and both ball and socket deformity, I had surgeries in infancy. What results is significant hip pain, arthritis, and the eventual need for a hip replacement when I can no longer manage the pain. All of this makes any type of exercise difficult. Additionally, genetics play a role in my obesity, as I suspect it does with many of the women who visit your practice. PCOS patients tend to struggle with weight gain. I saw my weight increase significantly with birth control use. While I admittedly love to eat, I do maintain a relatively healthy lifestyle and remain as active as possible — for an obese person with a physical handicap. Yes, I take an estrogen receptor pill. My oncologist didn't offer much of a choice. She told me it was the best way to prevent an estrogen-fed cancer from growing. She told me she did not anticipate that I would have any side effects. She told me that there are few usual side effects, if any. She was not concerned about increased risk of uterine cancer due to the use of that particular drug. I have faith and trust in my oncologist, and take the prescribed dosage daily.

So, back to the office visit. After telling me I was obese and taking an estrogen receptor pill, putting myself at greater risk for uterine cancer, he told me that next year he will perform an endometrial biopsy. He held his pen up in the air and pointed to the inkwell, trying to try to describe the diameter and length of the instrument he would use. With that, he ended our talk and took me to the exam room.

I was frustrated and angry. Where was the compassion I expected from this doctor I adored fifteen years ago? Where was the *"how did you handle the chemo? The radiation? How is your family? How are you?"* Nothing. Absolutely nothing. Fortunately, I am a stable individual *(although you may question this as you read my words).* My year was more than a little rough, but I was embraced by the love of family and friends, and enveloped in the prayers of many. I got through this awful year and came out on the other side even with a smile on my face. Where was the *"Hooray for you"* from this doctor who should be concerned about every aspect of my care? I complained to my nurse and shared my frustration about the doctor. She smiled gently and continued to take my blood pressure. I told her if my blood pressure was elevated it was the doctor's fault. I could tell she was uncomfortable and I felt that I should never have put her in such a position complaining to her. To be honest, I needed to talk to someone. I felt certain if I didn't express my dissatisfaction to her, I would have been furious when he re-entered the room. In fact, I almost walked out after the consult and had to talk myself into staying for the exam. I don't know if she shared my comments with him, or if he overheard us talking, or if perhaps he realized that he had lacked compassion, but he entered the room a different person.

At that moment, the doctor decided to ask me how I handled the chemo. He asked if I had felt a lump. He asked a couple of other things, but to be honest, I'm not sure what he said… because at the time he decided to be nice to me my legs were already in the stirrups, sheet above my knees, and my nakedness made the talking seem awkward. My answers were one-word answers, and I sensed he was aware I wasn't very happy with him.

After my exam, he decided to spend more time talking to me about the endometrial biopsy. He showed me the instrument. When I questioned if there wasn't a less invasive procedure *(remember, I have been poked, prodded, squeezed, biopsied, cut open,* stuck with needles, infused with chemo drugs and radiated this year), he said "yes, an ultrasound, but it would be a vaginal ultrasound. It costs more and it's a bit of a hassle." Okay. So, let's just get this straight…..the first option includes something similar to the inkwell of a pen only significantly longer being inserted vaginally and as he told me "hurts more than a pap." *(I wondered what it might feel like being inserted into a penis, but I didn't want to suggest that…yes, my sense of humor remained intact after chemo, too)*. The second option would be a vaginal ultrasound. *(I had those during pregnancies. They were uncomfortable but not overly painful)*. Expensive *(not to sound callous, but I have good health insurance)* and a hassle *(for whom might I ask is it a hassle, and why?)*. As a patient, I don't believe I was really given much of an option; and as a cancer patient, I have learned that I need to be my own advocate.

And the words that bothered me almost the most…

When the doctor asked if I had felt a lump, I indicated no, I had not. There was no palpable lump. I do self-exams at home regularly. My mammography technician did a thorough breast exam and did not feel a lump. My surgeon could not detect lump during examination. My cancer was completely detected by routine mammogram. The doctor told me I was **lucky**. I was offended.

I am not *lucky*. I am proactive about my health and go for routine screenings. A routine screening saved my life. Instead of telling me I was lucky, he could have and should have reinforced the importance of routine screenings. But, he told me I was lucky.

When I visited the hospital not once, but twice for surgeries, I didn't feel lucky. I felt scared and frustrated.

When I was told that my cancer was highly aggressive, I didn't feel lucky. I feared the worst.

When I had a medi-port fastened to my jugular vein, I didn't feel lucky. I felt terrified.

When I felt the pressure in my chest as my port was accessed, I didn't feel lucky. I felt sorrowful that I didn't have better veins, and disappointed that my prescribed chemo could cause tissue damage if infused through traditional IV.

When I watched bag after bag of chemo drip into my body, I didn't feel lucky. I felt tired, nauseated, and sad.

When I could eat nothing but Italian ice for ten straight days after chemo, I didn't feel lucky. I felt like a person who would do anything possible to remain hydrated and avoid a return visit to the oncology office for fluids. I lost 10-15 pounds in the ten days that followed chemo. But post chemo, I ate cookies – so I'm still obese.

When chemo gave me diarrhea and I had to take anti-diarrheal medicine, I didn't feel lucky. When the anti-diarrheal medicine made me feel constipated, I didn't feel lucky. It was one vicious cycle of diarrhea and constipation – followed by my fair share of nausea and vomiting. I didn't feel lucky. I felt like a sick person – a very sick person.

When all of the above had me zapped of all energy, I didn't feel lucky. I returned to the oncology office to have more fluids and medications infused into my veins. I felt exhausted both physically and emotionally.

When I had radiation tattoos and permanent marker drawn all over my chest, I didn't feel lucky. I felt like a permanent reminder of my illness would always be with me. Permanent marker eventually fades. Tattoos do not.

When I had to breathe through a snorkel type mask on the radiation table to protect my heart, I didn't feel lucky. Lucky would be snorkeling in the Caribbean. I suspect the doctor knows what it feels like to be lucky.

When my skin became raw and I had to dress my wounds with gel packs and lotions, I didn't feel lucky. I felt like the cancer treatments were never going to end.

And then, came a time for healing – a time for celebrating and feeling as normal as a post-treatment cancer patient can possibly feel. It was time to make all of the routine appointments I had missed in the last year (doctor, dentist, opthamologist, gynecologist, and the list never seemed to end.)

During my illness, I was surrounded by excellent health care professionals. I was treated as every patient should be always treated, whether they are a cancer patient, or not. I suppose this excellent care spoiled me a bit, and I expected nothing less when I visited your office.

One of the things I liked best about Dr. #1 was that one of the first questions he used to ask at the start of every visit was "How are the kids?" He had prescribed my infertility drugs, so I think he felt a little proud of my awesome family. I loved giving him the *annual report* about the wonderful little people in my life.

I would have loved to have a 30-second opportunity to tell today's doctor about my youngest daughter that he delivered into this world. She lives in a happy little bubble and it was her tender and youthful personality that helped bring normalcy to our lives during my illness. She is an A-student, a talented gymnast, and made the Varsity cheerleading team as a freshman *(difficult to do at our high school).* She is kind, loving, and compassionate. She avoids drugs and alcohol (*also difficult to do at our high school*) and is consistently respectful to adults. She, along with her two older siblings (*and my husband*) took excellent care of me during my illness, often putting my needs before theirs. They are certainly the reflection of all that is good in this world.

Dr. #1 also used to ask about family life in general. It was during a visit in my early 30s that I told him about my mother's Stage 4 colon cancer diagnosis. He immediately recommended that I go for a colonoscopy screening. I am now 48 years old and just scheduled my fourth colonoscopy procedure. Dr. #3 told me that in a couple of years, I should go for my *first* colonoscopy. *Whoops.* I guess he didn't review my chart. Teachers have a hard time respecting those who don't do their homework...

It's hard to leave a place you have gone for 23+ years, so I have some decision making to do in the next year. Whether in your practice, or somewhere else, I will find a doctor that is compassionate. I will find a doctor who recognizes that sometimes there are causes that contribute to obesity more than just a pile of cookies. I will find a doctor who believes in the importance of estrogen receptor pills post-cancer, and can better explain how significant the side effects may be. I will find a doctor who understands that I am not just lucky — I am a fighter. I fought like hell this year, and I'm not going to let the insensitivities of a doctor knock me down.

In many ways, things worked out in my favor. My cancer had not spread to lymph nodes. My cancer was Stage 1. I may someday, after all of this, be called cancer-free. But it was never, ever without a fight

I am hopeful that someone in your personnel office reviews letters carefully, and I am hopeful that my concerns are addressed. While every patient deserves compassionate care, sometimes the cancer patients need a little extra consideration.

I apologize for the length of my letter, but it's a little hard to explain something to those who haven't walked a mile in my shoes. I am not simply *lucky*.

I would expect that your office would attempt to follow up with me in some way. E-mail is my preferred method of contact. I can be reached at...

The wisdom in this story: No one should ever be afraid to be their own advocate for better care. And someone should invent a pen like instrument for the male anatomy. If one has already been invented, I think my doctor needs to be tested.

Doctor Office Update

Monday, July 25

My friends felt certain that I would receive a prompt reply from my doctor's office regarding my letter expressing dissatisfaction. I felt certain they would stamp it with the word *NUTCASE* and place it in my patient file. When I had not received a reply after eight *business* days, I sent it again.

I received an immediate reply: *I just wanted to get back to you. I did receive the letter you sent regarding your visit. I apologize for not getting back to you immediately. There is a process that I need to follow and I have not completed this yet. I hope you understand this. I will get back to you as soon as I am able. (patient advocate)*

Seven business days later I received another e-mail: *I showed your letter to one of the providers and also to Dr. #3. We are sorry that you were dissatisfied with your visit. Unfortunately, the correspondence between the patient and the provider does not always go the way the patient feels it should go. I am sorry that you have breast cancer and I feel for everything that you have had to endure over the past year. We hope that you will continue with our practice but also understand if you decide to transfer. We have several other providers that you can choose from for further appointments. If I can be of further assistance, please let me know.*

My reply: *This response is pathetic. I am not looking for your patronizing apology that I have breast cancer, but rather an acknowledgement that your doctor's manner in communicating with a patient was less than satisfactory. If the "correspondence between the patient and the provider does not always go the way the patient feels it should go," a good doctor would find a way to remedy that. A simple e-mail from an advocate who seems to be covering for a physician's lack of compassion is insufficient.*

The wisdom in this story: I'm not the nutcase. They fail.

266

The Beach

Monday, July 25

I stretch back in my chair and let the summer sun warm my face. The cool ocean waves cover my toes on this ninety-something degree day. I don't wear a swimsuit, but rather a cotton t-shirt and shorts to protect my radiation-sensitive skin. I worried I would be too warm, but the gentle ocean breezes feel lovely. A hotel towel *(I know, you're not supposed to take the hotel towels to the beach)* is draped gently over my chest to cover any spots my t-shirt and sunscreen may have missed. Even if for just one day, I am in my happy place. My family has always loved the beach, and this is a place where laughter fills my heart. I look to my right and see the hands of a man digging deeply into the sand. Those hands, my son's hands, sweep through the sand with same motion as when he was a toddler. While not elaborate, he is making a castle — with a moat...*always a moat.* He smiles as the waves wash in and stay long enough to fill the moat with water, and sighs deeply when his structure collapses. He runs off into the ocean, just in time to grab and dunk his youngest sister under the waves. She squeals, *even though my children know how much I dislike squealing.* She wants to appear angry, but the squeals are really pure delight, as she relishes in the attention of big brother. She pleads her case with me, and of course I need to intervene and tell him to stop, all the while laughing under my breath knowing moments later he will dunk her again. And he does — *again, and again, and again.* My middle child rides the waves for a while, and then retreats to her beach chair and becomes engrossed in a book. She is my reader. Teachers always strive to instill a love of reading in all children, and it secretly delights me to know how much this young lady loves to lose herself in literature. Eyes fervently focused on the text, she doesn't see that a huge wave is upon us, and gets sand and water in her eye. She of course blames this all on big brother, as he was blocking her view of the impending wave. I remind her to blink and allow the tears to flow, but to try not to rub her eye. After a moment or two, she is back splashing in the waves, the water spotted book tucked safely in her bag. And now, they are all in the ocean, my husband, too. 1-2-3-4. I count heads and then allow my mind to wander a bit. What a year it has been. During treatments, I never would have imagined that my energy levels would return to the degree that they now have, and I never would have imagined that I would be spending a summer day on the beach. This is my happy ending—*for now.* The pills, appointments, and scans that will fill the days ahead seem insignificant. The fear of recurrence of cancer will always be with me, but today I feel more normal than I have in a very long time. 1-2-3-4...I'm counting heads again. *How many years have I spent watching out for everyone's safety while at the beach?* As my four loved ones bounce in the waves, I listen intently and yes, above the sea sounds, I can hear their laughter. What a joy! And then I laugh a little to know that I am still counting heads of those who are much better swimmers than I could ever dream to be. Oh, I can swim, and swim quite well—but I have always been a bit intimidated by the ocean. Realizing that my constant head counting isn't really necessary, my eyes wander across the beach where I discover an adorable family. Mother and Father seem to be relaxing under the beach umbrella, and the children are with grandparents at the edge of the ocean. Grandpa chases after and giggles with the young boy, who appears to be about three, while Grandma holds on tightly to his older sister. Their eyes never leave their grandchildren, except for the small glimpses my way as I share in their joyful moments and our eyes connect briefly. Soon, a wide-eyed little girl who proudly tells me she is four appears beside my chair. She is collecting seashells, and she has noticed the bright smile of my daughter who has joined me on the beach. Her own family seems to be oblivious to her presence, and I say a silent prayer of thanks that they at least had the sense to have her wear a swim vest. She shows me her shells, but seems more interested in my daughter. She reminds me of the attention-seeking children I sometimes meet in my classroom. The ones who just need a little extra love. She comes and goes, and with each new shell we ooh and aah, and all the while her own family still doesn't really acknowledge her. She is beautiful. A blessing. I am glad that my daughter and I are on this beach to appreciate her. I look back to the other family, doting grandparents and delightful grandchildren. *I know what kind of grandma I want to be someday.* So many times, I have wondered what I will do if my cancer returns. Through tears I have told my husband that if it does, I may tell no one. I may not have the energy to fight the fight again. But then I realize, these are the days worth fighting for — *always.* God knew that I needed a little more time to settle the sibling squabbles, wipe the tears from the seawater splashed eyes, and love the ones who just need a little extra love. And as my son told me shortly after diagnosis, I need to be here to someday babysit my grandchildren. Like the ocean, cancer intimidates me. But like the moat around my son's castle, I am surrounded by faith, family, and friends. I have collapsed, but day by day, I am becoming strong again.

The wisdom in this story:

Grow old along with me,
the best is yet to be…

Michele's e-mail:

jellydonutdays@gmail.com

These are a few of my favorite things:

www.apple.com *excellent customer service*	www.mcdonalds.com *I recommend the McFlurry.*
www.broadway.com *Keep a show tune in your heart.*	www.pandora.net *My cancer bracelet is beautiful.*
www.disney.com *May all your dreams come true.*	www.peanutizeme.com *Create a Peanuts character.*
www.dunkindonuts.com *I recommend the jelly donut.*	www.puffs.com *I recommend Puffs Plus Lotion*
www.greenday.com *Have the time of your life.*	www.rachelplatten.com *Incredible inspiration….*
www.kleenex.com *Show you care.*	www.southwest.com *Sunshine is the best medicine.*
www.lifeisgood.com *Attitude is everything.*	www.verabradley.com *Compassionate customer care…*
www.loveyourmelon.com *gives hats to cancer kids*	www.victoriassecret.com *Buy PINK!*

Coming in September 2017

CHOCOLATE DONUT DAYS
Life after Breast Cancer, Cherishing Every Single Day

"It's just— I thought she'd always be here."
"In fact, she is. She is on every page you write."

(from Finding Neverland)

Publication Date: August 5, 2016
Fifteen years ago today, I lost my best friend.

35065711R00162

Made in the USA
Middletown, DE
18 September 2016